# THE
# DEMISE
# OF MEDICINE

ANDREW MORTON, MD

# THE
# DEMISE
# OF MEDICINE

The Terminal Diagnosis of American Health Care

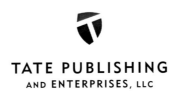

**TATE PUBLISHING**
AND **ENTERPRISES**, LLC

Published by Tate Publishing & Enterprises, LLC
127 E. Trade Center Terrace | Mustang, Oklahoma 73064 USA
1.888.361.9473 | www.tatepublishing.com

Tate Publishing is committed to excellence in the publishing industry. The company reflects the philosophy established by the founders, based on Psalm 68:11,
*"The Lord gave the word and great was the company of those who published it."*

Published in the United States of America

ISBN: 978-1-62854-849-5
Medical / Health Policy
13.08.21

# Contents

# Foreword

Eye-opening, disturbing, and timely all aptly describe Dr. Andrew Morton's first book. It is a deeply personal, yet widely appealing journey through the modern American medical system from the perspective of an actively practicing family physician. Tracing his development from an EMT to a medical student to a battle-hardened veteran of the Iraq war has given him wide exposure and experience that is reflected in his sometimes inflammatory, but always fascinating story.

From illustrative examples from real patients, to dealing with insurance companies and regulators, to revealing wasteful costs and practices, this reality-based story from a dedicated but often frustrated doctor offers guidelines for coping with and reforming a problematic and often seriously broken system.

This book is must-read for patients, medical professionals, or anyone concerned about the current state of medical care in the United States.

—Gerald D. Ramsey, Ph.D.

# Introduction

If you're expecting this to be a feel-good romp through the wacky adventures of a family physician, this really isn't your book. Let's face it—health care in America is broken. From the very basic organization of modern health care delivery to the financial structure, liability, all the way down to the office visit, the system is a dysfunctional mess. If you don't want to take a hard and honest look at modern medicine from a primary care physician's perspective, then put this book down and go watch television. After all, would television lead you astray? I haven't heard much discussion about defensive medicine, the effects of the high cost of insurance on your health care options, or the rampant problem with prescription drug abuse on my local channels. One may say, "I've seen all the doctor shows. I watch the news. I vote. I know what's going on in the health care industry." The issue is that the real problems in health care are the ones no one talks about. It's the big pink elephant sitting on your chest slowly crushing the life out of you that everyone pretends not to see. Or possibly you are having a heart attack. If it's the latter, I recommend you call an ambulance.

If you are currently breathing, and let's hope so lest the zombie apocalypse is upon us, then the health care system has affected you and will continue to do so until you are dead. Continue on, and some of what you read here will upset you. I hope it does. The industry of medicine has upset me for years now. If you've ever been to the doctor, saw one in passing in the hallway, or watched one (real or imagined) on TV, then you already have a perception of who we are, what we do, and how we behave. You may also have some conception of how the industry of medicine works. Hold that thought. It's not what you think.

It's much worse.

Consider this to start: The art of practicing actual medicine, the ongoing grind of what I do every single day often to the detriment of my personal and family life, is nothing like the media, the politicians, or even the lawyers would have you believe. It is not in reality tied to some ethereal code of ethics and morality. It is not glamorous. I do not show up in scrubs to a television show and talk to you about which supplements you should or should not be taking. I don't jet off to some developing nation to discuss water sanitation. And no, I don't live in a big house and play golf on Wednesdays. As a matter of fact, my day is mostly focused on survival—both yours and mine. Let me clear up some misconceptions for you.

Oh sure, everyone in the health care field has horror stories and doctor jokes. However, I'm not compiling a collection of campfire stories told late at night around the heart monitors, eating whatever the nightshift nurses brought in for the birthday pitch-in. I don't pretend to have the monopoly on anecdotes, but I will share my personal experiences with you. I will also share my opinions—personal, professional, and occasionally unprofessional—with you. Of course others will invariably disagree with me. I tell my patients that if you were to put ten doctors in a room and ask them a question you will walk out of that room with eleven different opinions. That is the beauty and the curse of the "art" of medicine. Some may not like what I am about to say.

A profession is defined as a "disciplined group of individuals who adhere to high ethical standards and uphold themselves to, and are accepted by, the public as possessing special knowledge and skills in a widely recognized, organized body of learning derived from education and training at a high level, and who are prepared to exercise this knowledge and these skills in the interest of others. Inherent in this definition is the concept that the responsibility for the welfare, health and safety of the community shall take precedence over other considerations."[1] We physicians as a "profession" have a reputation to uphold. I argue that we should have defended the profession of medicine long before I started practicing. A "job" on the other hand, is "a piece of work, especially a specific task done as part of the routine of one's occupation or for an agreed price."[2] The profession of medicine has become the industry of medicine, and my calling but a job. Those who define themselves by their occupation may feel that it is unprofessional to point out the flaws and pitfalls of the system; it's too late now to be indignant. This only contributes to the problem.

Personally, my first name isn't Doctor; it's Andy, and unfortunately I may have to find another line of work before my usefulness in the workforce is over. That may not necessarily be a bad thing; I live and breathe this crisis in medicine every day. Some days it's not worth it. This is real medicine, and I am on the front line. Here are my moccasins—slip them on and follow me for a few miles.

# Legal Disclaimer

As a general rule, I dislike lawyers. I think most doctors probably do. With the exception of my bestie's wife and my divorce attorney, everyone else is out of luck. Don't see me accepting your Internet friend request any time soon. There's a saying in medicine that goes, "It's not if you will get sued, but when."

According to a recent New England Journal of Medicine article, in America by the time a physician reaches retirement age, roughly 75 to 99 percent of all physicians, depending on specialty, will have had a malpractice lawsuit filed against him or her.[3] I'm a simple kind of guy. I guess it's the primary care in me. Let's average that number to about 87 percent. That's a pretty daunting statistic. If I had known before I applied to medical school that I have an 87 percent chance of getting sued, I might have reconsidered my profession. I spent over a decade of my life and bought the equivalent of a three-bedroom house in the suburbs just to have the opportunity to help others. In other jobs, employees may get a pin for years of service or maybe a set of cufflinks or a nice watch. I get a lawsuit.

Yes, I read the statistics, and statistics can be manipulated any which way to make a point. Some will rebut and say that also according to that article only 1 to 5 percent of all claims result in an indemnity payment and that I have nothing to worry about.

Others may say that the malpractice rate is only 7 percent per year. Sadly, as I will be doing this until I die, retire, or find a different job, that rate is misleading. If I only planned on practicing for one year, then that may be acceptable. However, I am still paying off my student loans, expenses incurred as partner in a physician practice, and of course, my children's college tuitions. I will therefore be doing this until I die or am no longer capable. That means that my lifetime personal risk of being sued is roughly 87 percent, thank you very much.

Let's dwell on malpractice a little more. I live in a small town with a population of roughly three thousand, and the county as a whole has about forty thousand residents. With the exception of my time in the military, I have always lived here and hopefully always will. If you listen carefully, you can almost hear whispers of John Mellencamp wafting down from the north on a warm spring breeze. We have a strong sense of community here. My children are active in school events and the community theater. I take them fishing during the summer, and we camp at the state park ten minutes from my home. I volunteer teach at the elementary school and am the appointed health officer for our county, as well the medical director for the volunteer fire department and nursing home. The community band plays in the gazebo on Friday nights from Memorial Day to Labor Day. My office staff has a float in the Independence Day and Halloween parades every year, and we have a booth at the county fair in August. Even though only about 20 percent of America's population lives in a rural community, I happen to be one of them.[4] I am happy here. Unfortunately, there's one aspect of country living that is not as pleasant.

In rural America we like to gossip. Most everyone is in most everyone else's business. It's the original reality TV but without the television. My neighbors probably know more about me than I do. Now let me present to you this hypothetical scenario: I see in the office Bob. Bob is married to Susie, who knows Betty.

Betty is married to Steve but is allegedly sleeping with Joe (Betty not Steve), because this is a small town and everyone knows that Betty and Joe are hooked up. They were seen at the church picnic talking together—that's a sure sign. Anyway, Steve knows a gal (because they actually are having an affair) who works at the county clerk's office who saw that Bob has filed a malpractice suit against me. Susie is an instructional assistant at the elementary school, and Betty works in the church office. We all understand from previous experience that Betty is a gossip; so right away we know this can't be good. At the end of the day Bob's lawsuit has resulted in Susie having hard feelings toward me and making my children's life more difficult at school while Betty's busybody nature has spread the word to everyone at church, which is a large portion of the town, that I "did Bob wrong," and if it were up to her then she would see another doctor. Got it?

Now this lawsuit, while probably frivolous and statistically only has a 1 to 5 percent chance of actually ending in any sort of settlement, would, if this were a true scenario, cause not only myself but also my family significant problems. Just trying to keep up with who knows what and how can make anyone's head spin, but it also has a direct impact on my ability to provide financially for my children. Out here the pool of patients is rather limited, both by sheer number of people available and by the fact that many are related by blood or marriage. Lose one patient, and I potentially lose an entire extended family.

Although this may seem extreme, it really isn't as far-fetched as one would imagine. Granted, this hasn't happened to me yet (knock on wood), but in my own real-life my recent divorce has created a similar effect on my patient base. People will naturally pick a side. Edward or Jacob? Hatfield or McCoy? Picard or Kirk? Whatever. Unfortunately in a small town every patient counts.

Another untoward effect of a lawsuit, even a frivolous one, is the psychological impact on the defendant, which in this case would be yours truly, Andy. Anxiety, depression, insomnia, and guilt are all common and prevalent symptoms following a mal-practice lawsuit.[5] Every decision I make is made with the intent that it is in the best interest of the patient, you, at that time. When there is a bad outcome, it's not only traumatic to you, the patient, but it is also psychologically devastating to me. Did I miss something? Is there something I don't know that I should? What could I have done differently? The doctor-patient relation-ship is just that: a relationship. Like any relationship, it goes both ways. To see someone that I have developed a bond with have something bad happen to him is difficult. To have that happen and then be slapped in the face with a lawsuit is heartbreaking.

What does that mean for this book? That means that although the situations and opinions are real, names have been changed to protect the innocent as they say (although we are not). We also have laws protecting the privacy of health information (not really, but we pretend). I prefer not to be sued quite yet if at all possible.

# Gallows Humor

There's a reason why medical jokes are funny. Humor is a way to disarm something threatening or unpleasant. It is a way to relieve tension, and it allows us to express anxieties. It's the ultimate coping mechanism, and shrinks will tell you it is also the healthiest psychological defense.[6] There's not much that's more unpleasant than pain, illness, suffering, and death. The medical profession delves into these topics at full speed with both eyes open, and for some of us ghoulish types it's actually pretty fun.

It is what I do for a living.

When I was a kid, just after the demise of Beta tapes and during the halcyon days of VHS, there was a pseudo-documentary that showed gruesome (for the time) images of death and dismemberment. I thought that was the most fascinating thing I had ever seen. As a matter of fact, I watched that movie until I had it memorized. My parents didn't appreciate it, and my friends just figured I would end up being a psychopath serial killer. Obviously they thought it was demented that anyone would think death and dying could be interesting. Perhaps no one at age fifteen should be wondering just exactly how high someone would bounce on asphalt from a fall out of an office building window—and I'm not necessarily disagreeing with that. However, it was the candid and honest way that it seemed to portray a topic that was mostly taboo in the 1980s that I found intriguing. As an adult, I have learned that there are many forensics books that discuss these topics. I can learn about the marks left from knife cuts into bone as well as the state of body chemistry immediately after death and the stages of larval growth on a corpse.[7,8,9] It's all quite scientific and a legitimate area of study. And even now, modern television is full of forensics shows making being ghoulish mainstream.

Rewind twenty-five or so years. Since just mentioning that movie creeped out my friends, I had mostly forgotten about it until one day when I was sitting around the lunch table with some of my fellow first year medical students. The topic of conversation was pretty much the usual stuff—life sucks; I'm going to fail my classes—and wondering why all the law students were already out of class. On this particular day amongst a heated game of euchre that we played to reduce stress and take our minds off of what we were supposed to be learning, the topic of conversation turned to death. Every classmate in that lunchroom had seen this movie, and, like me, most had memorized it. We had a great time reliving the suicides, the bear mauling, and all the other tragic accidents caught on tape. It was refreshing to be amongst peers who could have frank discussions about tough topics.

The other subject matter that everyone dances around is sex. It seems ironic that the two things that most of us do in our lifetime (have sex and die) are the two topics that we feel the most uncomfortable with. When I was in my residency in the navy, we had to rotate through the emergency room as first and second year residents. Every military base has three constants just outside the gate: pawn shops, tattoo parlors, and strip clubs. Someone has to supply the womanpower for the pole dancing, and generally it was the wives and dependents of the active duty members on base. They were also my patients.

One evening, probably three in the morning, a resident buddy of mine came back to the call room laughing. Of course we just had to know what was so funny. He tells us this story:

So there I am down in the ER. There's a gal being carried in by a couple of marines. The marines were very drunk but trying to act like they weren't. Her choice of attire made me wonder if she wasn't just a little bit cold, even though it was almost eighty degrees that night. I talked to her, and I find out that she's having ankle pain. "Okay," I say. "How did this happen?" She says, "I was walking across the stage in four-inch stilettos, and I tripped on my clothes." Given what she was currently wearing, I couldn't see how that was possible, but I get X-rays and, of course, she broke her lateral malleolus [leg bone near the ankle]. I put her in a removable boot and told her that she was off work for six weeks. She was upset, but only until she realized this happened on the job and this was a workers' compensation claim. She was going to get short-term disability.

My third year resident chuckled and followed up with this story:

So there I was in the ER. This young woman walks in complaining of vaginal discharge, so I do a pelvic exam on her. I put some of the aforementioned goo on a slide and added a drop of potassium hydroxide. I was relieved to not be overwhelmed by the odor of fish, performing the aptly named whiff test. Everything is so far so good at this point. I place a little more on a fresh slide for later. After finishing the exam, I went to the microscope to further examine the offending fluid. Bingo, there's your problem ma'am. Trichomonas are small microorganisms that are sometimes the cause of cervical discharge and inflammation. A half dozen or so were swimming on the slide. Bit of a nuisance these are. Not too horrible in the grand scheme, but annoying nonetheless. [They remind me of the microorganisms found in pond water that we used to look at in high school biology class.] When I go back to give her a prescription for antibiotics, she asks me out. I tell her that I'm currently unavailable, but I jokingly say she could give me a call in ten to fourteen days after she finished that prescription.

Although sometimes brash and inappropriate, the ability to laugh at ourselves is one of the best methods we in the health care industry have to ameliorate what otherwise would be sometimes unbearable conditions mentally. Many of my patients are also lifelong friends of mine or the parents of my friends or my former high school teachers. Sometimes I have to sit down with them and tell them that they have cancer and are going to die soon. That is not something that I relish. They look to me for guidance and support and hope, but sometimes it just isn't there.

Most recently I attended the funeral of the mother of one of my closest and longest friends. She was also my patient. I stood before her casket looking down at her resting there, and I thought about everything that had transpired over the past six months and the pain that my friend was currently experiencing. Was this my fault? What could have I done differently?

I do agree that it does get easier over time. That doesn't mean that it ever gets easy. Some may find gallows humor distasteful, crude, and offensive, but I find it vitally important and necessary, so when I ask you to hop on the table so I can check under the hood, I mean that in the nicest possible way.

# The Hippocratic Oath and You, A User's Guide (or Apparently, It Was a Stupid Idea)

The Dalai Lama has once been quoted as saying, "Our prime purpose in this life is to help others. And if you can't help them, at least don't hurt them."[10] In a nutshell, the Hippocratic Oath can be summarized in this one phrase: "Primum Non Nocere—above all, do no harm."[11,12] Amongst my many tattoos is that exact phrase, and assuming I have a mirror or am feeling extra limber, I look at it daily. It's my mantra, my motto for daily living, and in general just a really good idea.

The Oath also has subsections which, while staying true to core concept of primum non nocere, apply to specific circumstances that are just as true now as they were in the fifth century BC. Unfortunately, it seems that in modern American medicine we have taken the Hippocratic Oath and summarily tossed it into the trash.

The first concept of the Oath is to respect those who taught us and teach future generations what we know. That's pretty straightforward; share your knowledge. As a physician, it is my duty to teach. Most of what I do on a daily basis is teaching others. I teach patients about diet and nutrition. I teach about lifestyle choices. I teach about disease and disease prevention. I teach about medications and how they work. I teach nurse practitioner students, and I teach medical students the hallowed art of my profession. Most of this is word of mouth. I do not write textbooks, and I do not publish scientific journals. My charge is to educate about the core principles of medicine. Healthy choices, hygiene, lifestyle modification, and preventative medicine are staples. Having a discussion specifically about which chromosome the gene for breast cancer lies is not really relevant to my day. It may be important, but if that patient doesn't do self-breast examinations or come in for mammograms it's pretty pointless.

One would think that education and the dissemination of medical knowledge would be simple. However starting in the 1500s with royal grants given by Queen Elizabeth, the concept of intellectual property was born. This idea really took off with the British Statute of Anne in 1710 and the Statute of Monopolies in 1623, which are the origins of copyrights and patents respectively.[13] Now it seems that just about everything medical is copyrighted, trademarked or patented, and usually marked up in price about 300 percent of what it's really worth.

One day I found a medical supply catalog on my desk. It was big and bulky and reminded me some of the old Sears catalogs my parents used to get in the mail near Christmas that I would scour for things that I thought I wanted but could never afford. I flipped though this particular catalog, and my eyes landed on the crash carts.

A crash cart is a wheeled cart that stores medicine and equipment used in medical emergencies. If I need to incubate someone because they have stopped breathing or shock their heart back into rhythm, that's the cart I go for. The price tags on these particular models were in the range of a thousand to two thousand dollars each. After all, they were made of high-grade steel with rolling wheels and a five-year warrantee. Oddly to me, they also looked not so vaguely familiar. Also on my desk was a sale flyer for a local hardware store. They were selling a high grade steel tool box on wheels with a five-year warrantee that looked familiar, no, exactly like, the "crash cart" that was in the other magazine. These were on sale for about forty dollars. When our office finally did buy a new "crash cart" box, it sold at a sporting goods store for about fifteen dollars. It was plastic but had a nice carrying handle. It also fits spinner-baits and assorted lures very nicely.

If the most basic and fundamental principles of medical knowledge were being discovered today, it would most certainly be restricted to the point of unavailability. Everything from medications to medical equipment, DNA, and even amino acids and their subsequent proteins are patented now. Peer-reviewed medical journals in theory allow the exchange of new information and clinical research. However, even this is not free. The lack of adequate, and free, information will soon frustrate anyone trying to do research using PubMed. Expensive association fees or journal subscriptions ensure that someone is restricting widespread use, and I figure probably making a profit on the exchange of medical information. Unfortunately this is not limited to the medical profession as illustrated by the music industry's lawsuit Metallica et al vs. Napster, Inc. If there's a buck to be made with intellectual property, then we as Americans are after it. In this case I guess future generations of disenfranchised youth better pay up.

The next concept of the Oath is to practice medicine in accordance with your ability and judgment, which translates to "don't do things beyond your scope of practice." In other words, to be perfectly blunt, if you don't know what you're doing, don't do it. Dr. Conrad Murray was the physician convicted of involuntary manslaughter in the 2009 death of Michael Jackson.[14] This is not an isolated incident. Increasingly, physicians are being criminally prosecuted for medical care. Examples of these prosecutions include at least three obstetricians convicted of manslaughter or second-degree murder, a Colorado anesthesiologist convicted of reckless manslaughter, an anesthesiology resident charged with involuntary manslaughter, and an Oklahoma surgeon convicted of involuntary manslaughter.[15] Medical malpractice has now crossed over into the criminal court system.

If one of my patients has a bad outcome and there is an untimely death, not only do I have to worry about a malpractice suit, I now have to consider that there may be criminal charges pressed. I could actually be charged with murder. With that thought in the back of my mind, I sometimes find making the hard decisions that I need to make very difficult. It is easier to continue running expensive tests or continue futile and painful treatments or refer to other specialists for their opinion even though I already know the answer. The health care responsibility buck needs to stop at the family physician. There should be no one second-guessing that decision. I know you better than anyone else. I know you literally inside and out, but if I am going to be charged with mur-der, or even malpractice, because I was "negligent" or didn't "do everything possible," then I am going to avoid that at all costs. I like you, but I am not going to jail for you. Unfortunately and ironically, that mentality of "do everything possible" is not even in your best interest. Your last few months in this world may very well be filled with painful biopsies, expensive and futile treat-ments that makes you sick, and you will spend your last days hooked up to wires and tubes in the company of strangers rather than at home with your loved ones. Go figure.

This is a slippery slope. There are many risk factors for coro-nary artery diseases, which ultimately can lead to a heart attack.[16] These include such things as family history, gender, and age, which cannot be controlled. There are many other risk factors that can be controlled. These include high blood pressure, high cholesterol, diabetes, obesity, stress, smoking, and lack of physical activity. Will I be charged with a criminal charge if my patient refuses to eat better, exercise, lose weight, and take his medicine then has a heart attack and dies?

This isn't as far-fetched as it may sound. Payment structures from the insurance industry are currently transitioning from what is considered episodic care to performance-based care.[17, 18] The current "episodic" system is one in which a physician sees a patient and then is paid for that office visit. That is the same system we use when we call a plumber. The bathtub drain gets clogged, leaving old soapy bathwater to sit un-drained in the tub. Before the EPA comes in and declares it a wetland, you call the plumber. Joe comes over and snakes out the hairball causing the problem, the tub drains again, and you pay the man. You are happy; he is happy. Your coronary arteries become clogged—you call the cardiologist. He snakes out the french-fry grease from your artery. Blood flow returns to the heart. You are happy; he is happy. Pay the man.

Oh, but it's not that simple. In the performance-based model, we know through research that it was lack of exercise, too many fries, and a two pack a day menthols habit that caused the clog in the first place. As a primary care physician, I will soon become paid by ensuring that my patient's cholesterol is in range, he quits smoking, his blood pressure is under control, and he hits the gym. This is called "pay for performance" or "value-based purchasing."[19] In this payment model, physicians, hospitals, and medical groups are rewarded for meeting certain performance measures for quality and efficiency. Conversely, disincentives, such as eliminating payments for negative consequences of care (medical errors) or increased costs, have also been proposed. My specialty academy states: "there are a multitude of organizational, technical, legal and ethical challenges to designing and implementing pay for performance programs."[20] One of these, of course, is the liability for a negative outcome. After all, even though I cannot make my patient get off the couch and exercise, will I still be held accountable when he has the "big one?" What is the liability for a negative outcome? Is it not getting paid, getting a malpractice suit, or having criminal charges filed? I don't know, and I don't really want to find out.

In this profession, today, I can be held responsible for the death of another even though I was doing everything I could to help them. Those things happen. We are all human, and sometimes errors occur despite our best intentions. Regardless, if physicians stayed in their comfort and ability level, maybe we could decrease morbidity and mortality associated with direct physician care. In regards to the malpractice system, I am not saying that there should not be a process in place that identifies and removes "bad" doctors from practicing medicine. Lawyers will tell you that there aren't enough malpractice cases and that the rewards are insufficient to compensate for a lifetime of dismemberment or accidental death. Adverse events occurred for 3.7 percent of patients or nearly 99,000 New York hospital patients in 1984. More than a quarter of those adverse events were due to negligence. It is also reported that for every doctor or hospital against whom an invalid claim is filed, there are approximately seven valid claims that go unfiled.[21]

We need common sense in regards to malpractice. Just because you can do something, such as sue for negligence, does that mean you should? What is the downstream consequence of breeding an environment based on fear of retribution rather than the pursuit of good? The health care system in America should be nurtured and supported, not tapped on the nose with a rolled-up newspaper. I'm not a bad dog that just piddled on the floor. I'm the guy who was up all night taking care of your mother in the intensive care unit, but then the following day made a small mathematical error on a medication dose because I am tired, not because I am intentionally trying to hurt someone or am undertrained. If am doing everything I can to help others and I make an error, does that warrant a lawsuit? Criminal charges?

What is my incentive as a provider of primary care to continue doing this job then when I could do something else, like jet off to a third world country to discuss water sanitation or peddle nutritional supplements on television? Since 1900, the average lifespan in the United States has increased by greater than thirty years; twenty-five years of this gain are attributable to advances in public health and decreasing childhood mortality. During the early 1600s in England, life expectancy was only about thirty-five years, and the average life expectancy in Virginia colony of colonial America was only twenty-five.[22] Since 1900, infant mortality has decreased 90 percent, and maternal mortality has decreased 99 percent.[23] Should we bite the hand that takes care of us when we are sick, and keeps us alive when we would otherwise die? Without medical professionals and public health, where would we be? How many of you reading this now are over twenty-five? Due to an illness as a child, I would not be here today if it were not for modern medicine. I do not feel that I am entitled to the "compensation that I deserve" but am instead grateful for what others have done for me.

If I don't know something, or I make an honest mistake, I try to be the first to admit it. It's my experience that honesty is appreciated more than arrogance, but I guess sometimes that isn't enough. The increasingly disturbing trend that I see is a seeming increase in legal advertisements. If you take this medicine and suffer any number of potentially unrelated problems, call us, and we will see if you have a chance. Let's sue the doctor or hospital and see if we can walk away a millionaire. There's no penalty for trying. You don't have to pay them unless they win your case.

On any given day I can give you an example of both extremes of Hippocrates' tenant of "don't do what you aren't qualified to do." One day I had a patient that I received on call. He had apparently broken in to the local nature center and tried to steal the timber rattlesnake on display. The snake had other ideas, however, and bit him on the forearm. He presented to the medicine floor with an arm swollen and painful. Treatment of a rattlesnake bite, although unusual where I live, is not something foreign to me.

My training in the navy was excellent. I ordered antivenin and the appropriate supportive care. He improved over the course of a few days, and I eventually sent him home without any problems. I was asked a half dozen times if I was qualified to take care of this. I reassured all that this wasn't the first time I treated this, and yes, I did know what I was doing.

Another example that didn't turn out as well as I would have liked was a patient who presented with burns after a fireworks accident. His mother arrived on scene and, to her horror, he was not receiving the therapy she thought he needed. I work in a rural hospital and trained in a hospital with limited specialty access. I thought treatment was appropriate for the resources that I had on hand. Regardless, she was quite displeased, and within short order after her arrival to the hospital, he was whisked away in a helicopter to get "proper" treatment. Was I practicing out of my scope of medicine? She certainly felt so. I, on the other hand, did not. I weighed the risks and benefits of treatment, threw in my personal experience, and came up with a solution that I felt was acceptable.

Unfortunately in medicine it's not what you know or don't know that will cause problems, it's what you don't know that you don't know that could kill someone. And in this situation, it may well have been that the "standard of care" was different in this area than the standard of care that was taught to me.

The next tenant is don't abuse the doctor-patient relationship for your own personal gain. In other words, the exam room isn't a dating arena/sales platform. Unfortunately since the beginning of daytime television on through our primetime now, the allure of the handsome (and presumably financially well off) physician has been present to titillate the imagination. Patients routinely quiz me as to my marital status. For me it's usually Grandma trying to hook up her granddaughter, but sometimes it's the patient herself. My standard answer is no. I am working, and we need to keep it there.

Unfortunately, not all adhere to this philosophy and will abuse the relationship. I would like to think there's a special seventh level place for people like that besides jail. There's enough sexual predation in the world; physicians don't need to add to it. Unfortunately, it does occur in the health care field as evidenced by these headlines: "A Pasadena dentist who offered to reduce a female patient's bill in exchange for a sexual favor was charged with solicitation of prostitution."[24] Or the even more horrific: "A Delaware pediatrician accused of molesting more than 100 of his patients was sentenced Friday to serve his lifetime in prison."[25]

So, to recap, unless it's a friendly hug, please don't. Touch is an important part of the interchange between a doctor and the patient. I promise you I will find the sorest spot on your body and push on it. That's my job; that's what you pay me to do. Also, Grandma can hug me until the cows come home if that makes her feel better. I'm not talking about that kind of touch. You know which kind I'm talking about. I'm talking about the kind they discuss in the kindergarten orientation brief, the kind that makes me want to take a hot shower with lye soap. It's cute if it's you're an eighty-year-old grandma. Even if you're an eighty-year-old grandma looking to score (yes, that does happen) it's still pretty cute, I'll have to admit. Otherwise, it's just annoying. Let's assume for a moment that you are supermodel hot. Even if you were, there's nothing I could do about it except go home and cry into my pillow. I took an oath for a reason. Save me the angst. You don't want your doctor to go home and cry into his pillow. Most of the time, however, we're not talking lingerie photo shoot with a hangnail. It's usually, "Doc, you're cute. Do you mind looking at my rash? Maybe we can go out sometime." Okay, people, eww. I'm just saying. I have a hard time shifting gears and separating the concepts.

I will keep what I learn about people secret. Wow. That doesn't even apply anymore. In 1996, Bill Clinton signed into law the Health Insurance Portability and Accountability Act or HIPPA.[26]

This policy meant to improve the efficiency and effectiveness of America's health care system by encouraging the widespread use of electronic data exchange. Wonderful in theory, but what it really did was free up the constraints that protected your health records in the first place; namely, the doctor's offices. Granted, the system of paper charts kept by physicians were cumbersome, inefficient, and contributed to the duplication of many services such as lab and diagnostic testing, but at least your information was more secure than it is now. Due to requirements placed upon my office by the Centers for Medicare and Medicaid Services (CMS), we are now on an electronic record system. With just a couple of keystrokes I can export all your embarrassing little secrets out to any format I wish: the web, a zip drive, fax, e-mail, you name it. And now thanks to HIPPA, I can do this without your knowledge or permission. I recently downloaded an entire medical record and e-mailed it to a patient at her request. What's keeping that information secure? Federal law? Facebook privacy policy? I think not. Ponder the following:

Directly cut and pasted from the Health and Human Services website (hhs.gov) is the following:

Individually identifiable health information is information, including demographic data, that relates to:

- the individual's past, present or future physical or mental health or condition,

- the provision of health care to the individual, or

- the past, present, or future payment for the provision of health care to the individual, and that identifies the individual or for which there is a reasonable basis to believe it can be used to identify the individual. Individually identifiable health information includes many common identifiers (e.g., name, address, birth date, Social Security Number)."

It goes on to say:

A covered entity is permitted, but not required, to use and disclose protected health information, without an individual's authorization, for the following purposes or situations: (1) To the Individual (unless required for access or accounting of disclosures); (2) Treatment, Payment, and Health Care Operations; (3) Opportunity to Agree or Object; (4) Incident to an otherwise permitted use and disclosure; (5) Public Interest and Benefit Activities; and (6) Limited Data Set for the purposes of research, public health or health care operations.[18] Covered entities may rely on professional ethics and best judgments in deciding which of these permissive uses and disclosures to make.

So basically as I read this, almost anyone, at any time, for "public interest activities" (such as the church picnic, I suppose) can learn that you were last treated for gonorrhea three weeks ago after your return from what you described as a "business trip" to your wife and colleagues. Hello, big brother, and good-bye, privacy. The lawyers love this law and request medical information all the time, as do insurance companies digging for reasons not to pay your medical bill. I see a half dozen such requests a day on my desk. I have no choice (it's the law, after all) that I send them the requested information. Failure to do so may result in civil and criminal charges. Do I notify you or ask your permission? Absolutely not.

Now, that's not to say that I'm going to spill the beans any time soon to your next-door neighbor. That's tacky. Even in a small town that's tacky. What you are doing and with whom is really none of my business to begin with unless you are dating my daughter. Besides, I do try to adhere to the standard of the Oath I took when I earned my degree. I probably won't remember what you told me after you walk out of the exam room anyway. I examine almost five hundred people per month, which means that it all runs together after a while. I usually don't remember whom I just saw twenty minutes ago. Were you the one with the broken foot or the erectile dysfunction? If I really wanted to know I would just refer back to your chart (I can do that; I don't have to remember). When I walk out of the office after fourteen hours of dealing with sometimes difficult or unstable people, the last thing I'm dwelling on is your colonic health, so don't ask me about it at the grocery store. As long as everyone is getting better and nothing is missed medically, I'm okay with not remembering your test results while I am shopping for milk and bread.

The Hippocratic Oath specifically states that I will not give a lethal drug to anyone nor do anything to cause an abortion. Roe versus Wade pretty much shot down the latter in 1973, and lethal injection is currently the most common form of execution in the United States. [27, 28] Someone has to administer that medication, and I'm pretty sure it's not the janitor. Jack Kevorkian also tried to convince us in the 1990s that assisted suicide of the terminally ill is an acceptable form of medical treatment.[29] I deal with terminal illness on a daily basis. It is part and parcel of being a family physician. I see every manner of pain, from cancer pain to the emotional pain of having someone you love slowly forget who you are, to the pain of watching a spouse wither and die or a child pass suddenly and unexpectedly. Too many times I have to look a person in the eyes and tell them they have cancer. For many that's a death sentence. Last week I saw a patient who wasn't feeling well. He looked like he didn't feel good. I had been with him and his wife when she battled lung cancer. It was a long fight, and eventually she died. It was obviously difficult emotionally for him since he loved her dearly. It was difficult emotionally for me as well. I was with them throughout the diagnosis, treatment, and her decline and death. I was with them when they decided to stop treatment. I took care of him and was with him when he arrived with his new wife a few years later. Now he himself has cancer. He does not want treatment; he saw what his previous wife went through, and he doesn't want his new wife to suffer the way he did. Now I have to have the difficult discussion with him. Do we attempt to treat his cancer with the hopes that we can extend his life another six months to a year for his new wife, or we do not and watch him die quickly?

Every day that I am alive on this planet is, in my opinion, a good day. Some days are better than others, but I appreciate each one. Death comes too soon for many as it is, and for others who are in insufferable agony not soon enough. It is my job to comfort, to help both the patient and the family when and how I can, whether through the administration of medications, counseling, or just being present in the moment and listening. "Modern" medicine seems to be obsessed with doing everything possible to extend life. This often comes at the expense of the patient and family, both financially and emotionally. My experience has taught me that many families of a dying loved one often don't want "everything possible" done; they just need someone to tell them that it's okay to let go. However, I don't feel it is my job to take a life. The time and the place are not mine to decide.

# Training

Why am I a doctor? In a nutshell, it's because I didn't want to be an electrician.

It's the 1980s. Gas prices are at the ridiculous amount of $1.12 a gallon. Some band called Guns and Roses just released an album called *Appetite for Destruction*, and Metallica still represented the disenfranchised. My first car was an '82 Subaru with a bad CV joint.

In the sticks there's not much industry. Unless you are a farmer, the expectation is a commute to work. My father, being no exception, drove fifty miles one way into the city to work as a maintenance electrician for a box company. He had five different jobs from the time I started paying attention until his untimely death due to cancer. He worked seven days a week for as long as I could remember, and yet we never lived above the national poverty level.

I became very familiar with government social programs. One rare day when I was about fifteen, he and I were fishing and talking about the usual things fathers and sons talk about in those circumstances. We came to the topic of occupations. He told me that under no circumstances should I be an electrician, especially a maintenance electrician. It was miserable work and harder to find each year as manufacturing was starting to go overseas.

Fast-forward a year. I am trying to figure out what I want to do with my life. I typically scored very well on any standardized test I took in high school, so I figured I was probably smart enough to find a job that didn't require too much manual labor. Putting up hay and doing seasonal farm work as a teenager taught me the value of a good education. I wasn't made to go pick cucumbers for the rest of my life. I wanted to work smarter, not harder, as they say.

I'm in high school study hall. In walks the army recruiter. It was a wonderful presentation. The Cold War was in full swing, and it was our job to stamp out the Communist threat. Oh, and you can earn money for college. Bingo. I'm in. Where do I sign? There was no other way I was going to college unless I could find a way to pay for it myself.

The Armed Services Vocational Aptitude Test (ASVAB) is a test administered in high school to determine military vocational potential.[30] As I filled out my paperwork at the Military Entrance Processing Station (MEPS), a soldier stood over me with the dubious honor of pigeon holing me into an occupation, thus sealing my fate in the army. He looked at my ASVAB score and told me that I would do wonderfully as an electrician. I thanked him and told him that no, that was not what I wanted to do. He then proceeded to offer me a job as an infantry medic. I would do well there also, he informed me after looking at my scores again. The propaganda video he showed me looked pretty interesting, so I signed up as a medic, although I didn't know quite what they actually did besides run around with a stretcher and look important.

Let's talk about training. I mean, it's easy to be a doctor. Just ask anybody. On a given day I hear any number of the following:

"Sally down the street is a nurse, and that's just like being a doctor. She knows as much or even more than that doctor I saw the other day."

Or "I just looked up my symptoms on the Internet, and it told me what I had and how to treat it. I don't know why I have to pay someone to write me a prescription."

And of course, my favorite, "I have this buddy who has a friend who had something just like this. He ended up having [fill in your favorite horrible disease here]. I'm sure that's what I have."

In my early days of working in health care, I had the opportunity to experience a range of responsibilities starting at the tender young age of eighteen. I had just finished the army infantry medic course at Fort Sam Houston, Texas. The civilian equivalent of this is an emergency medical technician (EMT) or ambulance driver. My first practical civilian application was in our local hospital as a tech in the emergency room. I would work three twelve-hour shifts a week. I won't lie to you; it was fun. I had the opportunity to change dressings, clean wounds, get vital signs, and all other sorts of "important" things like that. I felt that without me slathering that abrasion with antibiotic cream, the patient just might not make it. It was very easy for me to get lost in the hubris and feel that my role in patient care was more important than it probably actually was. In addition to having four days off a week, the other beauty of that job was I had a role that was needed, but I didn't have any real personal responsibility. If I didn't know how to do something or didn't feel like doing it, I just wandered over to the closest nurse, played stupid, and passed the buck. At the end of my shift I clocked out and was out of there until next time days later. What the patient's outcome was really had no relevance to my day. Whether the patient lived or died made for great talk around the nurses' station, but I had no personal or professional stake in it.

Fast forward again. I just graduated with honors from the infantry medic school at Fort Sam Houston and for the most part liked what I did on drill weekends. It's now my freshman year of college. It was school policy that each and every freshman had to meet face to face with a counselor to declare a major. Since my parents had not gone to college, I didn't even quite know what declaring a major meant.

Counselor: "So what is your major?"

Me: "Um, I don't know. Do I have to pick now?"

Counselor: "No, but it helps."

Me: "Oh. I don't know."

Counselor: "What do you want to do when you grow up?"

Me: "Have a job and work."

Counselor, sighing: "Well, what do you like to do? What are you good at?"

Me: "Um, I don't know. I like being a medic for the army. That's pretty fun."

Counselor: "Oh, okay. So you're pre-med then. You might as well get a biology major as well, since they're about the same."

Me: "Okay. Can I change it if I want?"

Counselor: "Sure."

Being pre-med also meant that I was automatically a member of the pre-med club. I tried going to a meeting once. Between you and me, that was way too intense. There was entirely too much tension in that room. I couldn't take myself that seriously. I wanted to hang out—not make diamonds. As the son of a poor electrician, I couldn't relate to the offspring of third and fourth generation physicians or some such silliness. Maybe if they handed out secret decoder rings or something I would have stuck around. After that incident I declined to attend any further gatherings, but I did get a flier in my mailbox once a semester or so that had important "pre-med club" information.

Physician training is significantly more involved than keyword searching the Internet or classes at the local community college. Let's face it, we all know this on a superficial level, but

I don't think we all actually understand it. One of my greatest frustrations with this profession is this point exactly: knowing something isn't the same as being able to appropriately apply that knowledge.

Medicine is more than being able to recollect facts. Anyone can Internet search and get more information in seconds than I could memorize in my lifetime. The ability to assimilate information and determine what is relevant and what is not, add in personal experience, and apply it to an individual patient is what makes a physician good at what he or she does. Maybe if we can all understand this we can better understand how the system in part fails. I don't want to bore you with the thought processes that I have to go through to come up with a list of possible diseases you have or your treatment options. It may be interesting to me, but I wouldn't expect you to care. Just realize that's my job to understand. How I think is less important than knowing that there are more than just isolated facts rattling around in my noggin; there's practical application of that knowledge. I don't care how specifically a mechanic fixes my car or how an architect draws plans to build a bridge, but it is important to me that Jim knows how to tear down a transmission so my car doesn't break down halfway across the bridge just as the poorly engineered support structures fail, causing me to plummet to the icy river below.

If the system is working properly, then knowing how I think should be irrelevant to everyone but fellow physicians. Rather, understanding that I am qualified to make medical decisions and deferring to my clinical judgment should be paramount. I dedicated well over a decade of my life just getting to the point where I am qualified to make decisions on a daily basis that do literally mean life or death. Unfortunately modern health care has so eroded that deference that for all intents and purposes I might as well have gone to McUniversity or saved my pennies and bought a box of caramel popcorn for my medical license.

# The Making of a Doctor

What exactly is the "health care system?" What is "medicine?" It is, on the absolute most basic, historic, and practical level, the evaluation and treatment of a patient by a physician. Let me repeat that. The practice of medicine is the evaluation and treatment of a patient by a physician. There will be a test at the end; please remember this.

Becoming a doctor made simple (as I have been trying to teach my children with varying degrees of success over the past few years) starts in high school. That may seem ridiculous, but it's significantly more difficult to get accepted into medical school if you don't get accepted into an honors program in college. That being said, lets assume budding doctor did well in high school and also graduated college with a bachelor's degree and good grade point average. That's four years of undergraduate education. Prerequisites include the life sciences such as biology and organic chemistry, and a fair amount of math and physics.[31] This isn't bunny level biology or pre-algebra, by the way. Also, per University of Louisville, courses in "paramedical school" such as pharmacy, nursing, or optometry do not fulfill the premedical science requirements. Okay, so far so good. That's all very achievable, and really in the grand scheme of things not at all special. I can only imagine that business majors, pre-law students, and

engineers all have similar requirements. I personally had the luxury of completing my four-year bachelor's degree in three and a
half academic years, thanks to George Bush Sr. and a little thing
called Desert Storm. My junior year spring semester was spent
getting shot at and patching shrapnel wounds on Iraqi prisoners
of war while my colleagues were presumably playing beer pong
and chasing nursing students, because that's what I probably
would have been doing.

Just prior to this moment, my first-hand introduction to
post-traumatic stress disorder, drill weekends in the army reserve
would consist of working at our local veteran's hospital. There the
care was significantly different than I was used to doing as a tech
in the ER. I was responsible for more comprehensive care on
sicker patients. This included care of chronic conditions such as
wounds and tracheostomies, which are those breathing tubes that
come out of people's necks. My first introduction to long-term
care was here. My very first day of work at the VA fresh out of
training consisted of changing dressings on a patient with bedsores with wounds that literally wrapped around his lower spine.
It was draining green foul-smelling pus that I learned later is a
bacterium called Pseudomonas, which is particularly difficult to
eradicate. I also had the pleasure of cleaning tracheostomy cannu-
las bright and early on Sunday mornings. These were metal tubes
shaped like the letter J that latched into a cuff on the patient's
neck so they could breathe through it. Usually these people had
large amounts of thick foul mucous clogging the trachs, and my
manipulation of their airways would cause them to cough snot
balls up through the hole in their neck and all over me. It was my
job then to soak the metal trachs in peroxide and scrub off the
funk with a toothbrush. It was then that I developed a healthy
disdain for anything mucous that I still have today.

I was in the army reserve during my formidable college years.
Yes, I fell for the "serve your country, earn money for college" propaganda of the 1980s. Be all I can be or whatever. It was certainly

worthwhile, and I still miss serving my country. Unfortunately for me at the time, my reserve unit was about one hundred miles from college. On drill weekends I would drive in and spend the night with nurse Bubba (before he was a nurse) for the weekend.

I first met Bubba in a refresher class for medics. Because I had enlisted into the army reserve three days after my 17th birthday, I had completed my basic training the summer break between junior and senior year of high school but had not yet gone to school to be a medic. As far as a soldier, I was in the club but otherwise untrained and pretty useless. They enrolled me in this class to keep me contained until I could finish training and be a productive member of the organization. I'm not sure why Bubba was there. He acted more like someone had put him in detention and he didn't want to be there. Regardless, I parked myself next to him simply because that was the only available seat left in the back and proceeded to try to understand what in the hell they were talking about up front. The instructor was jabbering on about the proper method for treating a sucking chest wound with plastic wrap and duct tape when Bubba leaned over to me:

Bubba: "Dude, wanna go rappelling after this?"

Me: "Okay." I had never gone rappelling before and really wasn't even sure what that meant. I didn't get out much.

Bubba: "I have the stuff in the trunk of my car. I know a spot where we can tie off to a tree. It's about eighty feet up."

Me: "Okay."

But after lunch the story was different.

Bubba: "Me and a couple of the girls from the unit are going out to dinner after this. Wanna go?"

Me: "Okay."

Not only did I not get out much, apparently I was easily influenced by others.

I immediately liked the guy. Although we didn't end up actually rappelling until some years later, it was, as they say, the beginning of a beautiful friendship. Bubba and I became inseparable. He was a sergeant at the time, and as such was my boss. He made sure I was squared away for drill weekends. I lived at his house when I was in town for drill, and he made sure my uniform looked sharp for inspection. That usually meant that he ironed my clothes himself, because I hadn't a clue how to iron and at eighteen didn't really care to learn. His civilian occupation then was tech for an adolescent inpatient psychiatric ward. He taught me how to interact with patients and communicate with them. He taught me how to care for patients as well as be caring.

During undergraduate, I again forayed into health care as a certified nursing assistant or CNA. In this line of work I helped mostly with what are called activities of daily living or ADLs. This includes going to the bathroom, getting cleaned up, eating, moving from the bed to the wheelchair, that kind of thing. I worked nights then because I was trying to learn biology, chemistry, and some other required but questionably unnecessary liberal arts stuff at the time. On the night shift, my workday started with having the pleasure of getting the residents cleaned up after dinner, which usually meant scrubbing them down after their afternoon constitutional. Then after that it's off to bed. If you're thinking of visions of snuggling down in their nice quilt with sugarplums dancing in their heads, think again. More like the fifth layer of hell in Dante's *Inferno*. Wailing and gnashing of teeth, rolling out of bed, crying, you name it. And thanks to the well-meaning Omnibus Budget Reconciliation Act (OBRA) of 1987, psychotropic medications are limited in residents of long-term care facilities.[32] Oh sure, less people are falling and breaking hips or twitching uncontrollably, but when the demented patient who won't stay in bed tries to claw your eyes out when you try to redirect them toward the boudoir, a little nighty night pill would sure be appreciated. Finally, once everyone is appropriately tucked in for the evening, then time for a horrific amount of charting. After that, another round of bottom checks, then time to turn them over for the umpteenth time. We don't want them to cook too long on one side. That's how we wind up with bedsores that I would have to subsequently clean and change dressings on the next week at the VA hospital. The night ends with more paperwork, then off work until the next night when the process starts all over again. Lather, rinse, repeat.

Oh yeah, I almost forgot. They're heavy. You wouldn't think Grandma would weigh so much, but "not quite dead" weight is really pretty heavy. I can't rightfully call it dead weight because dead weight gets wheeled away in a cart with nice big wheels on it. Everyone else is technically still alive and thus hand delivered. They have lifts for "biguns," but it's not really practical for everyone else. Takes too long to set up; there are too many people to flip and turn and no time to do it. There's never another person to help, so single person lifts on an octogenarian built for two isn't the smartest idea but is usually the norm. Backaches and sore muscles were standard for me. I have a very healthy respect for those who do that day in and day out. I'll pass, thanks.

I never really saw any happy nurses when I worked at the nursing home. At the time I never could really figure that out. After all, they weren't lifting from the commode to the chair or cleaning up Old Lady Jenkins for the tenth time that night. They just seemed a miserable bunch. I decided then that nursing wasn't the profession for me. I wasn't sure why they all looked so angry, but I knew that whatever the reason I wanted no part of it.

One particularly crappy Sunday morning at the VA hospital, I was in the middle of my second tracheostomy care. It was way too early in the morning. I had been up most of the night with Bubba hanging out with my army buddies and was in no mood to clean funk. As I stood there retching like a dog after a crabgrass salad, scrubbing off thick white mucous with my trusty toothbrush, I happened upon a wondrous sight. In bounced three or four youngish individuals in crisp white lab coats. They snatched the chart from the bitter old nurse, popped their heads into my patient's room just long enough to see what I was doing, poked a bit at him, listened to his chest, and they were out the door. They barked a few things at the nurse, jotted a note in the chart, and they were down the back stairs quicker than they arrived. I was in profession heaven. I wanted that job. Screw changing nasty wounds, worrying about catching some horrendous infection, and hurting my back. That was the job for me. This epiphany came to me the tail end of my sophomore year of college. That was just before I had to take my MCAT.

One random day the flier I received from the pre-med club informed me that I needed to take the MCAT. I wasn't sure what that was, but I registered for it anyway. I didn't have a back-up plan with regards to what I wanted to do with my life at that point. I was mostly finished with my biology major, and unless I wanted to teach high school or get a different degree I was still pretty unemployable. Maybe this medicine thing wasn't so bad after all. I don't think I ever saw an unemployed physician, not that I really knew any physicians to begin with, but that was beside the point. At the bookstore I found a review guide for the MCAT. I took it home and flipped though it while watching the new episode of *Star Trek: the Next Generation*. The following day was the examination.

The Medical College Admission Test (or MCAT) is our admissions examination that we take in our junior year of college.[33] Imaging combining all the science learned in all the classes since kindergarten and then taking a final examination on it, incorporating that entire fund of knowledge plus problem solving skills. Oh, and you have to do well on it, because you are competing against everyone else in college who wants to get into medical school.

Then there's the interview.

Shortly after receiving my scores, I received a letter saying that I should schedule an interview for medical school. That sounded reasonable, so I borrowed a collared shirt from my older brother (I didn't have any dress clothes of my own, couldn't afford any), wore dark pants, trying to hide the fact that they were jeans, and off I went. I stood in line with about fifteen other interviewees. They looked nervous. More importantly to me, they were all well dressed, suits with ties and all. I suddenly felt really out of place.

The guy in front of me was wearing a charcoal three-piece suit with matching tie. He seemed awfully confident, I thought. Thirty minutes later he comes out. His eyes were puffy, and I think I saw a tear as he sniffled past me. Was he crying? Oh, wow. What kind of interview was this? I was about to find out. I walked into the room and sat down. There were two desks at opposite sides of the room and some crusty old fellows in white lab coats sat at each desk. They instantly started quizzing me on my application, each firing off questions one after the other. It was much kinder than being screamed at by opposing drill sergeants like I had been exposed to previously, so I thought it was rather entertaining:

Interviewer #1: "So why do you want to be a doctor."

Me: "Because I like it, and I think I would be good at it."

Interviewer #2: "Are you committed to being a doctor?"

Me: "Um, I'll do the job, if that's what you mean."

Interviewer #1: "What are you going to do if you don't get in to medical school?"

Me: "It never crossed my mind that I wouldn't get in."

Interviewer #2: "Hypothetically, what will you do if you don't get accepted?"

Me: "I guess hypothetically I would have to go back to school or teach high school biology since I'm not really qualified to do anything else."

Interviewer #1: "Your grades are okay, but I see you dropped out a semester your junior year. I'm concerned that you aren't committed to medicine."

Me: "Oh, that. I didn't drop out. My army unit was activated. I was in Iraq."

Interviewer #2: "What did you do over there?"

Me: "Infantry medic. I did the usual stuff. Bullet wounds, shrapnel, sick people, whatever."

After that the rest of my interview degenerated into me waxing sentimental about Desert Storm. On the way out they both thanked me and told me that they hoped to see me soon. I walked out of the room wondering why Three-Piece-Suit Boy was blubbering. They seemed like nice enough fellows. The interviewee behind me looked at me as I tossed my leather jacket over my shoulder and walked away. I just shrugged at him in the "beats me" kind of way and went home. Two weeks later I received my early acceptance letter.

My first two years of medical school were spent reading as much as I could for as long as I could. Studying for medical school has been described as like trying to take a drink of water from a fire hose. There is too much information, and it is presented very quickly. A typical day for me was arise at four a.m., read until class at eight a.m., then home at five and read until midnight. The weekends were nicer, because I had a full eighteen hours of reading all at once on Saturday, but only twelve hours on Sunday, because I had to take break. For some of the classes I only had enough time to read the course material once before being tested on it. This is the beginning of our indoctrination into the lifestyle of medicine. And of course, at that time, I had a new wife and an even newer baby at home. I'm sure that didn't add to my stress at all.

I had the fortune of going through medical school the same time that Bubba was going through nursing school. When I would spend weekends at his house just for giggles we would swap textbooks and compare notes. After all, they're basically the same, right? He described the difference between nursing school and medical school using an analogy that I think is very appropriate.

Imagine that you are a mechanic. Now imagine that you have a book that is describing a car. Your book shows you pictures of round things, and tells you that they are tires. It tells you that the tires are used to help propel the car forward. There are usually four tires on a car, but there can be more or less depending on what type of car you have. The tires are made of rubber. Sometimes the tires need to be changed, and it would go into some detail about how to change that tire. This would be a nurse's textbook.

My textbook wouldn't have a picture of a tire on it at all. It would have the chemical structure of the rubber used for the tire and how it was manufactured in detail. It would have a blown-out view of a steel-belted radial labeling the inner liner, the carcass ply, beads, sidewalls, crown plies, and tread. We would have to know the tire speed rating and the tread life, and be able to recognize the tread pattern between an all-weather radial and a performance tire.

My last two years of medical school consisted of learning the art of information gathering. It consisted of learning how to gather information from the patient, how to gather information from the chart or tests, and how to present it in some sort of coherent, logical format. It also built upon the basic science that we were taught in the first two years of school and showed how this information was relevant to actual people.

Occasionally we could, if we were good, actually touch a patient or assist with a procedure such as hold a surgical retractor or take out skin staples. Keep in mind that at this point I have completed six years of education and passed the first of four certification examinations before being allowed to actually touch a patient in any meaningful way. I suppose the medical school wanted to make sure we actually knew something before we jumped in and manhandled people. Realize that's equal to or more education than most every other fully completed medically oriented program including nurse practitioner, physician assistant, or pharmacist. Hold that thought.

The last two years of medical school were also clinically oriented, which means we emphasized patient care more and classroom lectures less. I rotated through a different specialty of both medicine and surgery monthly, learning the basics of that specialty. We also did most of the "scut" work (that's Latin for "to whip") for the rotations that were hospital based. For these inpatient rotations I would, at some unholy hour in the morning (previously in college this would normally be the time I would be rolling home and into bed) collect the vital signs and results of labs or diagnostic tests, present the patient's condition to the residents, and mostly just try to make sense of everything. This was our transition between academic education and clinical application. Even what the residents were learning was nothing like I learned in my first two years. I was all about the Kreb's Cycle and energy production on a cellular level. I could look at a slide and tell you the tissue type and discuss what was happening on the cell membrane for just about any process you wanted to know about. I could discuss for hours the depolarization of heart muscle as it leads to muscle contraction. If you pointed to a body part I could tell you what it was, what it did, the nerve and blood vessel distribution of it and all of its neighbors, and all in Latin. Although this was important, there was so much more I needed to learn about actually managing a patient and his or her medical condition.

I also learned during this time that there were some aspects of medicine that I wasn't designed for. Standing still for twelve or so hours picking at tissue through a magnifying lens or instrumenting people's colons all day is not what I consider a good time. The physicians that do that for a living can have it; I will pass, thank you very much. I know what they have to do to earn their income, and they earn every penny of it. The sacrifice physicians make for the well being of others comes at a high price. What is a saved marriage or a weekend with your children worth?

My residency focused on trying to make sense of all the information that I learned in medical school and making useful decisions with it. My first year, or intern year, was spent trying to understand what was important and what wasn't. Namely, how I check the oil and what I do if the car is a quart low. If a nurse would call me in the middle of the night with a set of vital signs, I had to learn whether what she was telling me was clinically important or not. Is that blood pressure something potentially life threatening, or was it something that could wait until morning? If it is too high or too low, then how do I fix it? Why do I choose one medicine over another when they are in the same class? Is one better than the other in certain circumstances? Am I familiar enough with this medicine to prescribe it? What are the side effects and adverse reactions? What happens if the patient has a reaction to it? Am I prepared to treat that and if so, how? Is there an alternative to this medicine? Is the risk of taking the medicine higher than the risk of not taking anything at all? Stir in sleep deprivation and a schedule that encompassed about 110-hour work weeks. That first year was unimaginably stressful. As an intern, however, these midnight scenarios usually meant I asked either my upper level resident or the nurse herself. The nurses working with me at my teaching institution had seen a hundred scenarios just like this one and were good about pointing me in the right direction. They may not know specifically why something is the right answer, just that it is. They have been taught how to start the car, so to speak. It is my job to know what happens after the key is turned. Some things just aren't taught in textbooks, and without practical application and experience, medical knowledge is pretty useless. Although Dr. Google is great about providing information, he lacks the ability to provide you with sound medical advice that is specific to you. It may also be true that new "baby docs" don't know how to insert a urinary catheter or know the usual and customary steps for working up common medical problems such as fever or shortness of breath, but they can explain to you in excruciating detail the pathophysiology of just about anything you would ever want to know.

The second and subsequent years of residency are spent continuing to expand this knowledge. This is very specific depending on the specialty. For example, a general surgeon learns to cut and sew and an obstetrician learns to deliver a baby. By the time a doctor finishes his or her residency, he or she is more or less able to handle everything on a practical level that will be encountered in the real world. It is here that we learn the tools that we use every day. We learn to think like doctors.

Building on our fundamental knowledge base, we learn to treat common problems that we see every day, and we learn how to work through problems that we have never encountered. We are able to create a list of possible reasons why something is amiss. This is called a differential diagnosis and is, in my specialty, one of the most important tools that I possess with the exception of communication skills. If I am presented with a problem, I can mentally drill down to the basic cellular level and create a list of possible causes of this problem. For example, if a patient presents with leg pain, I can give you a significant list of things that can make your leg hurt. This could be due to something obvious, such as that broken bone sticking out through the pants. It could be due to a problem with the nerves, such as nerve damage or neuropathy from diabetes or shingles, or many other causes. It could be due to a blood vessel problem, such as swollen or varicose, inflamed, or clotted veins. It could be due to poor circulation called peripheral arterial disease or arterial insufficiency. It could be due to stretching of the skin from swelling, and then we delve into the subsequently large list of things that cause leg swelling.

It could be due to a problem with the bones, such as a nutritional deficiency or anatomic problem. It could be due to cancer spreading from a distant source. It could be from infection. It could not be coming from the leg at all. It could be phantom pain from a leg that is no longer there, referred pain from a spinal disorder, or "somatic" pain from an underlying psychological disorder. Even still, the patient could just be lying.

Once we have paired down this list to the top few possibilities, then we must learn the proper methods to evaluate and treat this. Is an X-ray indicated, or is an MRI better? Better still, should we stick needles into the nerve and measure its electrical conduction? Should we ultrasound it or check labs? All of these questions must be considered before the next step: officially diagnosing the problem.

Once we have the diagnosis, it becomes no less easy. There are many different ways to treat the same problem: lifestyle modification or medication, surgery or sympathy? Again, ten different physicians in a room will yield eleven different opinions. Each treatment is tailored to the individual patient. Can a patient tolerate a certain medication or not? If not, then what are my options?

My third year in private practice introduced me to a patient whom I will call Evan. Evan had multiple medical problems, which made his treatment quite complicated. One of his medical problems was inflammation of his stomach called gastritis. Any word with "itis" at the end usually means inflammation. His "itis" was particularly bad. Unfortunately, it was also very difficult to treat. He had been evaluated by specialists, gastroenterologists, who had said that if he didn't get his gastritis under control he was at very high risk of developing a bleeding ulcer, which could be potentially life threatening. The standard treatment for gastritis is medicine that decreases the production of stomach acid, which allows the lining of the stomach to heal. He had many other medical problems in addition to his gastritis that made him intolerant to most medicines. Some of these were allergies, and some were reactions to other medicines that he couldn't change because they were essentially keeping him alive. After significant trial and error, I found a particular medication that worked very well for him. It soothed his stomach, and it resolved his stomach pain.

Unfortunately, in his particular case, he was on Medicaid. His particular version of Medicaid would not pay for his medication. They stated that there were other medications that were covered in the same class as the medicine that worked for him. He could not afford to pay for the medicine himself, because he could not work, and his social security check only covered his living expenses. I tried to get this medicine approved through his insurance. I called the company, and I even wrote a long letter outlining his medical condition in detail. I specifically stated, "If he does not get this medication approved, he will die." It was still denied.

Three months after the final denial, Evan developed a bleeding and ulcer and died in the middle of the night at his home. I wish this were an isolated incident. Unfortunately, it is not. I see this same scenario played out again and again. I find it difficult and demoralizing trying to find alternatives for treatments that work simply because the cost of the medication or treatment is prohibitive.

Back to residency…

In residency, we simply tried to find practical applications to the basic science. Using the car analogy, I could tell you after medical school what a car was made out of, and I could describe a car to you, but I couldn't tell you how to change the tire or start the engine, and forget about driving the thing. At this juncture in our education the nursing profession has the upper hand in practical matters of medicine, and they know it.

I occasionally find as I'm flipping through magazines in the checkout line articles that address this very topic. Often I will see collections of anecdotes around seasoned hospital nurses "straightening out" naïve or arrogant residents. Although these stories are meant to amuse and in some cases enlighten, one must be careful not to think that they are the norm. Unfortunately, this attitude is becoming more and more prevalent to the point that the lines between what I do and what others in the "industry" do are indistinct. This is not necessarily to the benefit of anyone in the long run.

> When first the Fox saw the Lion he was terribly frightened, and ran away and hid himself in the wood. Next time however he came near the King of Beasts he stopped at a safe distance and watched him pass by. The third time they came near one another the Fox went straight up to the Lion and passed the time of day with him, asking him how his family were, and when he should have the pleasure of seeing him again; then turning his tail, he parted from the Lion without much ceremony.[34]

As with the Aesop fable, familiarity breeds contempt. The role and responsibilities of the physician are being slowly eroded by the media, the legal profession, and even other allied health professions. The tools we hone and more importantly the thought processes physicians develop to diagnose and treat are different than the tools nurses or any other medical paraprofessional use. Generally speaking they tend to learn through hands-on application and algorithms, whereas I learn through theory and an understanding of the basic science. This allows me to work through the problem and make a decision based not on the recommendations of an "expert" but on my own knowledge and logical thinking skills. After all, most "experts" do not have more formal training than I, just more experience. Also not every patient can be plugged into an algorithm. Not every patient is straightforward. I would venture to say that most patients are not straightforward and present unique circumstances that do not fit neatly into predetermined treatment plans.

# Slight Difference

This difference becomes glaringly obvious to me when I work with nurse practitioners, which is every day since my practice consists of six physicians and a nurse practitioner. Nurse practitioner training makes them think differently; with emphasis on prevention, education, and executing a care plan, not necessarily the diagnosis and treatment of a disease state.

Depending on the state in which they practice, nurse practitioners have varying levels of responsibility. In some states they function under the direct supervision of a physician, and in other states they work independently. My overall experience with these "mid-level" providers is that the education and training is not comprehensive enough to properly evaluate and treat patients independently. This is dangerous.

Briefly, a nurse practitioner is a nurse who has completed her bachelor of nursing degree and has gone on to complete a post-graduate program, either a masters or doctorate degree. The program focuses on the nursing model, which emphasizes holistic medicine, preventative care, and patient advocacy.[35] Unfortunately, my job as a primary care provider encompasses not only that but significantly more. Let's refer back to the car analogy for a minute. My concern lies in basic sciences and pathophysiology. A physician is trained in the art of understanding why things are happening, generating a list of possibilities (called a differential diagnosis), and treating based upon this list. A NP is presented with common scenarios and is expected to learn treatment algorithms without necessarily understanding the nuances of why they are doing what they are doing. They may know that for a patient with medical condition X they treat that with medication Y, but they do not understand what, on the cellular level, is happening.

The American Academy of Family Physicians describes the difference this way:

> Due to his/her seven years of medical and clinical training, a family physician can provide all the services of a nurse practitioner. But more importantly, the family physician brings a broader and deeper expertise to the diagnosis and treatment of all health problems, ranging from strep throat to chronic obstructive pulmonary disease, from unsightly moles to cancer, from stress headaches to refractory multiple sclerosis. The family physician is trained to provide complex differential diagnosis, develop a treatment plan that addresses the multiple organ systems, and order and interpret tests within the context of the patient's overall health condition…. Nurse practitioners are trained to recognize and treat common health problems, such as strep throat, ear infections and conjunctivitis. They are trained to monitor specific chronic conditions such as hypertension, high cholesterol, and high or low blood sugar problems. They provide preventive care such as immunizations. They educate patients about chronic conditions, medications, nutrition and exercise. They refer patients to the family physician when a patient has multiple symptoms that may or may not be related, a condition that is not specific to the nurse practitioner's training or a condition that has multi-organ effects and/or requires multiple medical interventions or medications. The nurse practitioner is trained to recognize and treat the three or four most likely causes of a patient's symptoms.[36]

This may seem unnecessary and overly cautious if you are the one trying to fill the primary care shortage that is expected in the years to come, but if you are the ill individual whose life depends on the nurse practitioner's ability to properly treat you and your specific situation, I would think that that difference would be very important. Unfortunately not everything fits into an algorithm, and not all problems present in a classic or "textbook" way.

In my office we have a meeting with the office management and providers on Friday. It is during that time we discuss issues, both administrative and clinical. Very recently my fellow physician brought up a topic of concern to the meeting. He passed out copies of a "wellness physical" that a patient of his had just received from a nurse practitioner at the local pharmacy clinic. This "physical" discussed smoking status, weight and exercise options, most recent cholesterol readings, his need for colon cancer screening, a discussion of healthy lifestyle choices, and he received his flu shot while there. It failed to address or mention at all any of the chronic disease states that this individual had. It failed to mention any past medical history ("none" was entered into that block) or acknowledge that this person was on multiple medications. It failed to take into account his cardiac risk factors or family history. It failed to address his uncontrolled blood pressure that he had at the time of the "physical." Had the patient followed the wellness guidelines as presented without taking into account his cardiac risk factors or his currently uncontrolled medical problems, he could have very well ended up dead of a heart attack or stroke.

This nurse practitioner was given the authority to "diagnose" and treat illness, or in this case perform a wellness examination, without being given the proper tools to do so. In my opinion to make the statement that a nurse practitioner working at the corner pharmacy "clinic" who has had probably six years of education at a level that is of significantly less detail than mine has the same basic fund of knowledge and therefore the same authority to practice medicine as I do after eleven years of education, is tragic and dangerous. This misfortune is self-perpetuated in the hubris of the nurse practitioner programs. They seemingly do not know what they do not know and self-regulate themselves by having separate certification examinations. It is my opinion that to practice medicine at the same level of a primary care physician, they should be held to the same standard. My recommendation would be to simply have all primary care providers with the same level of responsibility and authority, which may include physician's assistants in some states, take the same certification examination across the board regardless of educational background. This would ensure that all providers be able to "function" at the same level of competency. Ironically this would probably mean "dummying-down" physician certification examinations, but at least we would know roughly where the bare minimum of education lies. When I talk to a nurse practitioner that I do not know on the phone, I really have no basis to know that she even understands what she is talking about. Many times she cannot tell me what else is on her differential diagnosis or what else she could do to further rule in our out other potentially life threatening conditions, or even what the other possibilities are.

Before we get out the torches and pitchforks, let's think about this for a minute. Of course, there are multiple instances where physicians do dumb stuff too. I've seen it firsthand. I've probably done some of it. Being able to regurgitate information doesn't make someone a good doctor. There has to be insight and common sense also. I get that, but if the fund of knowledge is not there at the front end, then it will never be there after the fact. Also, my angst lies in the slow blurring of the lines between physicians and other allied health care industries. The term "health care provider" is becoming very prevalent in the general vernacular, and I have witnessed nurse practitioners with a doctorate degree (an academic degree, not a medical degree) referring to their own self as Doctor So-and-So.

To know what you do not know is sometimes more important than actually knowing something. If I have a clear understanding that there is some medical condition that I am not proficient at understanding—for example any number of relatively uncommon endocrine disorders, such as Conn's Syndrome—or I understand that for some presentation by a patient there may be a condition that I could be overlooking, such as Lupus, then I can adjust for that. My primary duty as a physician, after all, is to do no harm. I will gladly turf someone to a specialist if I am uncomfortable with the presentation or it involves an aspect of medicine that I know I am not good at. To not know what you do not know makes you dangerous. A family nurse practitioner is often on the front lines of patient care and will see the patient with multiple complaints and atypical (not textbook) presentations for illnesses. It is very important that they have a clear understanding of what they do and do not know. Although I do feel that there is a place for mid-level providers in our country, the independent practice of medicine without direct physician supervision is dangerous.

As the health officer for my county, I am responsible for not only the health department proper but also our maternal health clinic. In this clinic we have a nurse practitioner. In my state, she must have a preceptor (me) who audits a certain percentage of her charts as well as be available for consultation/guidance if a situation arises in which she is not comfortable. I was fully comfortable with this, until one day…

I am in my weekly meeting with the health department administrator and my clinical manager for the health department. We are going over the usual stuff that a rural health department has to deal with which, unfortunately, includes a shrinking budget with expanded responsibilities. On this particular day a situation arose that needed to be addressed:

Clinical manager: "I need to talk to you."

Me, thinking: *Oh, that's never good.*

Me, saying: "Okay, what?"

Clinical manager: "So we had a situation at the Maternal Child Clinic."

Me, thinking: *Ugh…what now?*

Me, saying: "Oh?"

Clinical manager: "We had a patient who came in with a blood pressure that was through the roof, and it wasn't addressed."

Me: "Go on."

Clinical manager: "We had a patient come in with a blood pressure that was 220/110, and it wasn't taken care of. The nurse practitioner released her without addressing this."

Me: "What happened exactly?"

Clinical manager: "We had patient come in for a routine examination, and while she was here was found to have this blood pressure. Because the nurse practitioner was only used to doing pap smears and pelvic exams, she either didn't recognize the significance of the blood pressure or wasn't comfortable dealing with it. She let the patient go without doing anything about it."

Me, thinking: *Ah, crap.*

Me, saying: "I think we need to find out exactly what happened, be sure that we identify all potentially life threatening conditions, and at the very least address them so that the patients are either started on appropriate treatment or referred to someone who can."

Me, thinking again: *Because if that patient goes home and has a huge stroke between now and the time she is seen by another provider, I don't have a legal justification as to why we didn't address this at her "preventative" visit. And guess who gets named in the lawsuit? Oh yeah, me…*

At the other end of the spectrum, a very good example of a difference in training that still works well clinically is the training between allopathic physicians (MD types) and osteopathic physicians (DO types). I am trained as an allopath. Practitioners of homeopathic medicine (to describe modern medicine) used this term historically as a derogatory word.[37] In the navy my family practice residency had both MDs and DOs. Generally speaking, there we defined the difference by saying that allopathic physicians looked at a "systems" approach to medicine, and each system (such as the respiratory system) was treated more or less independently. Osteopaths, on the other hand, are taught that each organ system interacts with each other, and the patient must be looked at as a whole. Osteopaths are also trained in the art of musculoskeletal manipulation.[38]

The ultimate outcome is that regardless of which training program a physician underwent, the licensing and certification examinations are the same. A family physician with osteopathic training has to demonstrate the same level of competency as me—whether they feel that musculoskeletal manipulation is beneficial or not is none of my concern. I know that at least on the most fundamental level they have the same knowledge base as me. One might even make the argument that I have the inferior training compared to an osteopath. Definitely the osteopaths that I trained with were certainly very bright and knowledgeable and knew more about the interaction of organ systems than I. If a nurse practitioner feels that she should have the same rights and responsibilities as I, then she should be held to the same level of knowledge and competency.

This also extends to other professions who feel that they possess the knowledge and skill set to adequately diagnose, treat, and manage medical problems. As reported by Daniel Weiss, Senior Editor of pharmacytimes:

- The country's largest association of medical doctors has come out against expanding the role of pharmacists in prescribing medications.

- The American Medical Association's House of Delegates has adopted a policy against allowing pharmacists to prescribe medication without oversight by or an order from a physician.

- The FDA argues that the move would help improve access to needed medication for many patients, but the AMA has countered that the proposal could jeopardize patient safety.

- In order to ensure that patients receiving medication under the new paradigm would be properly diagnosed and monitored, the FDA proposal raised the possibility of employing technology as well as expanding the role of pharmacists. For example, patients could access diagnostic technologies at a pharmacy or via the Internet, and pharmacists could perform routine monitoring using diagnostic tests and determine whether a patient should take a given medication. [39]

Not surprisingly, many pharmacy organizations showed support for this proposal, but they emphasized the importance of receiving higher incomes in exchange for the added responsibilities. In a perfect world I would love to only see one problem per patient. The concept that individual disease states can be "carved out" and treated independently of the patient as a whole is naïve. I am routinely treating multiple problems simultaneously, because they all interact with each other. Will a pharmacist understand the delicate balance between kidney failure and congestive heart failure? In certain circumstances one must create one to solve the other. My experience is—probably not. I receive daily requests from pharmacists requesting me to adjust a medication or discontinue a medication because of what they perceive as an adverse reaction or potential adverse reaction. It is my job to take that into account and come up with a solution that will benefit the patient as a whole. I am not discounting the knowledge base of a pharmacist has of medications, but knowing how a medicine works is only a small part of what I do.

Here's another simple example that I see very commonly. A patient with a serious infection presents to my office. They have an allergy to penicillin. They also have allergies to some other common antibiotics, or the organism growing is sensitive to only a certain class of antibiotics called cephalosporins. I write a prescription for an antibiotic, cephalexin, and the patient takes it to the pharmacy. The pharmacist refuses to fill the prescription because there is supposedly cross-reaction with this antibiotic if someone is also allergic to the penicillin class of antibiotics. So my choice is: Allow the patient to take the antibiotic and watch them have an adverse reaction, or do I give them no antibiotic at all and watch something really, really bad happen to them? Which is the lesser of two evils? What is it here that we do not know?

The Western Journal of Medicine published in 2000 an article that I found very enlightening: It is a well-known "fact" in medicine that at least 10 percent of patients who are allergic to penicillin are allergic to cephalosporin antibiotics. [40] However, if one were to actually look at the research and understand the basics of how a biology lab works (again, how is the tire made?) we would notice that during the manufacturing process many early antibiotics were frequently contaminated with penicillin and, thus, people would have an allergic reaction. Also, due to the very nature of how we are made on a genetic level, patients who are allergic to penicillin are slightly more prone to be allergic to any antibiotic. So, when I send a penicillin-allergic patient to the pharmacy with a prescription for cephalexin, I warn them ahead of time what to expect and tell them to get the prescription despite the protests.

The FDA's proposal involves only maintenance medications that can easily be monitored. A pharmacist can not only prescribe the medication but monitor the labs as well. What, again, is the definition of practicing medicine? The argument is that this greater access to care would allow the patients the ability to receive their medications without the "usual frustrations" associated with a doctor's visit. Oh, boy. Those "usual frustrations" are called a history and physical examination, or if you prefer, medical decision making. People are not static. They change and quickly. Your state of health today is not was it was two years ago. Plaque builds up in the arteries, organs fail, and we all get older. I need to examine the patient, perform routine health maintenance, which includes but is not limited to the basic labs drawn for that blood pressure medicine. Again, what about abnormal labs that do not fit within the protocol, or are the labs isolated only to the disease state that was carved out of the patient? Is that isolated calcium level clinically relevant, or was it not even drawn? It certainly could be. A certain amount of basic general chemistry is standard practice. Many conditions only present as an isolated abnormal lab found incidentally. That's why we do basic blood work on an annual physical examination. Is that isolated elevation on the serum calcium hyperparathyroidism or worse a metastatic cancer? If patients routinely and exclusively see a pharmacist for routine medical care, will things such as these be missed? If so, who is liable? Will the pharmacist be sued for failure to diagnose, or will it once again fall back upon the primary care provider who hasn't even seen the patient for two years because he has been going to Walgreens? Are pharmacists trained to properly treat the patient's co-morbid depression? Are pharmacists trained to understand and identify the warning signs for suicidal behavior?

If this wasn't about money, why would pharmacy organizations be so eager and willing to take on more responsibilities? Limited NPs and physician assistants usually work in the same office as and under the direct supervision of a supervising physician who does chart audits, is available to answer questions immediately, and directs the treatment plan. Will an independent pharmacist (or independent nurse practitioner, for that matter) understand the clinical relevance of that vague discomfort that the patient described as he was walking out the door because it did not fit into his protocols, or will he allow a patient with unstable angina who is only a few hours from having a massive heart attack go home without proper evaluation and treatment? Do not think that these scenarios are "worst-case" or "extreme examples." This happens on an almost weekly basis.

# Para-Professionals
# and the Hero Mentality:
# My Experience with Heroism

The Dunning-Kruger effect is a mental bias in which less skilled individuals mistakenly rate their abilities as much higher as they may actually be.[41] This bias is attributed to an inability of the unskilled to recognize their mistakes. Charles Darwin once said, "Ignorance more frequently begets confidence than does knowledge." On the other hand, actual competence may weaken self-confidence, and those who are above average may not recognize the limits of their position or abilities.[42]

I once came upon the scene of an automobile accident with personal injuries. As I was bent over evaluating one of the victims, another bystander approached. He nudged me to the side stating, "I'm a nurse. I have this."

To this I replied, "When you get to the part where you need to call the doctor, I'll be over there."

I define the "paraprofessional" as someone who has just enough training to feel empowered to make potentially dangerous decisions. This makes them difficult to work with. This is in contrast to a professional, who works within his or her training and ability and in collaboration with the health care team rather than in spite of it.

I had a forty-something female that was having abdominal pain. It sounded like gallbladder disease for the most part. I wanted to get some basic labs to rule out other potential problems such as a misbehaving pancreas. I sent her to the lab and told her I would call her when the labs came back. A week passes, and I don't have her lab results. My assistant calls her to check up on her. She is still having pain. I ask her why her labs weren't done, and she tells me that because she had a mint in her mouth at the time she went to get her blood drawn, the lab tech refused to draw her blood. The tech said that the labs I wanted were fasting labs, and since she had a mint, then she wasn't fasting, and she refused to draw them.

Similar scenario, different patient: I'm worried about an acutely inflamed gallbladder, which can be a medical emergency. The patient had a glass of water a couple of hours before she went downstairs for her scan. I realize the gallbladder may be a little contracted in this situation and am prepared to deal with a suboptimal study. The ultrasound tech refused to do the test, citing that she would not do the test unless the patient had been fasting for six hours.

I was on labor and delivery. I had a woman who was in danger of delivering a preterm infant. I had stabilized her as best I could, but she needed to be transferred to a medical center with a maternal fetal specialist and a neonatal intensive care unit. I had neither. I had spoken to the specialist, and he was willing to accept her to his facility. We called EMS...and then we waited. And then we waited some more. Meanwhile, the patient was still contracting and was in danger of delivering a very preterm infant in a facility not at all equipped to handle that. We called again and asked what the holdup was. Apparently there was an unofficial "rule" that there had to be one ambulance that was not in use in the county in case there was an "emergency." The remaining ambulances were out on runs, and it might be a while until any of them returned. Apparently a preterm delivery was not, in their eyes, considered an emergency. When the EMS crew did finally arrive almost three hours later, the EMT taking the history decided it was his responsibility to take a long and detailed history of the patient, although my paperwork was complete and literally in his hand. After an almost forty-minute interview, he decided that she was "worthy" of transport, despite my protest that she was going to have this baby any minute if they just didn't hurry the hell up and get her out. But, of course, my opinion was of no concern—I was just the attending physician; they were in control.

It was Sunday morning. I had an elderly person who was complaining about lower leg pain. On examination the leg was cool and pale. I was concerned about obstructed blood flow to the patient's leg. I wrote an order that said I wanted an immediate (stat) ultrasound to evaluate the blood flow, and if it was abnormal then I wanted to be called. Monday morning, I find that the ultrasound tech refused to come in from home to do the ultrasound. Apparently she determined on her own that an arterial ultrasound study was not an emergency and refused to come in. Because my order said only call if the test was abnormal, the nursing staff did not call me to tell me the test was not performed. When I reevaluated the patient, the leg was dead. I transferred the patient to a tertiary medical center where the patient underwent a lower leg amputation, which might have been avoided.

I do admire those who will put themselves in harm's way for others, even if my apartment neighbor's oversized four by four truck with the mounted blue lights takes up extra parking space. I am neither a coward nor a hero; I am a survivor. As such, I understand that I am more useful staying alive than rushing off to this emergency or the other. I do not find milling about a fatal car accident rewarding or fulfilling by any means. I've seen enough death. I still see enough death. I just try to not be the cause of it. Let me share with you my Desert Storm as I described it in a thesis I wrote two years afterward (see Appendix B).

I joined the United States Army Reserve on 29 February 1988. At the time, I was a junior in high school. Because I was still in school, I went through basic training during the summer after my junior year. I then when through AIT (advanced individual training) at Fort Sam Houston, Texas as a 91A10-Medical Specialist, often called combat medic, during the summer of 1989.

I did not join the army because I was patriotic; although I am. I did not join because I really needed the discipline; although it helped. I did not join because I needed the adventure, because my life is one big adventure without having to search for it. I joined for only one reason. I joined for the college money.

I chose to be a medical specialist for a variety of reasons. One of which is that the course was short enough to take during the summer. Another is that I was thinking about taking pre-med courses and applying to medical school. At that point, I really had no experience with the medical profession, other than the rare visit to the doctor's office for the flu. No one in my family is a doctor nor even in the health care field. I thought that I needed a little contact with the field before making a choice, so I decided to be a medic. I would be gaining medical experience and be able to pay for school at the same time.

I graduated with honors from AIT and developed a passion for the medical profession. I worked at a nursing home for a few months during my freshman year, but due to lack of time and sleep, I had to quit and concentrate on school. During the summer of 1990, I worked as an emergency room technician at a hospital close to where I grew up. It was there that I really decided that I wanted to be a doctor. During my drill weekends for the reserves, I work on the surgical ward at the Louisville VA hospital. There, too, I find what I do rewarding, even though traveling from Muncie to Louisville once a month is very inconvenient.

In the autumn of 1990, Iraq invaded Kuwait. On January 26, 1991, about 9:00 a.m. on a Saturday morning, I received a telephone call that would change my life forever. At the time, I was here at Ball State in the second semester of my junior year. I had been in class for about a month. The call started by saying, "You are hereby ordered to active duty in support of Desert Storm." I would report to Fort Knox on February 1. Approximately three weeks later, I was in a foreign country wondering how close to the front I was going to end up. Unfortunately, I went all the way.

For me, this was a traumatic change. First of all, I was thrown from a liberal college campus setting into a very disciplined, rigidly structured organization with very little time to adjust. Secondly, I was put in a combat unit. Thirdly, I was alone. I was not a happy camper.

I had a very rough time the first few weeks I was there. In the military's overwhelming brilliance, the sent a reservist with absolutely no field experience to an armored infantry unit on the front line the day before the offensive. During drill, I usually work at the Louisville VA hospital on the surgical ward. While there I work as a corpsman, which is roughly equivalent to a nursing assistant. I take care of old, sick veterans. I wash them up, change their dressings, take their vital signs, occasionally start an IV, and mostly joke with them (provided they are conscious) until it is time to go home for the weekend and do it again the next month. The only field experience I have received since I graduated from basic is walking from my car to the hospital and back, which is every bit of forty yards or so. Of course, sometimes it is cold or raining, but essentially it isn't very taxing on me.

However, within a span of a couple of weeks, I had been literally dumped into a combat unit in the field. Now only was it a combat unit, it was an armored combat unit in the middle of the war. I was, needless to say, clueless. The first day that I got to my unit, I was directed toward a group of odd box-shaped vehicles on tracks and was told to go jump into that 113 until the 577 could come pick me up.

My reaction was: "Huh?"

They said, "Do you see that deuce and a half?"

"You mean that big truck?"

"Yeah. Now, do you see the Bradley behind that?"

"The what?"

"The tank-looking thing."

"Oh, that."

"Well, directly to the left of that is a small armored vehicle. That is a 113. A 577 is like that, only it has a larger top on it. Got it?"

"Sort of."

Of course that isn't exactly the conversation, but it was very similar to that. It got even worse later on, when we had to put up the camo netting, build a hasty fighting position, put up the tent extension, set up the medical supplies, or basically do anything. I was totally lost.

The transition from civilian to combat-ready soldier was also a mess. Without my book bag slung over my shoulder, I felt very awkward. I couldn't sleep in and skip the war if I wanted to. I was sleeping in the sand with the scorpions, not in my bed or any bed for that matter. During my first few days there, we moved constantly, so we were forced to sit on the track as it pressed onward, broken only by the occasional pop of an anti-personnel mine as it exploded underneath us.

The transformation from civilian to combat-ready soldier, such as the one I experienced, was a very difficult one. The change was literally an adaption from one society to another, completely different one. The rules were different, the lifestyle was different, the norms and values were different. For me, it was a transformation of personality. Expectations of me were different. I was supposed to know a certain amount of medical knowledge, and this knowledge, or lack of, might mean the difference between life and death for some of those men. I have training equivalent to a civilian emergency medical technician, but I had no experience with most of medications that we had, and that was a major part of the job. I had no knowledge of a lot of what I was expected to know out there, because I was never exposed to it—ever. It was not taught at AIT, and I did not learn it during drill weekends. As a student (biology/pre-med) I was not exposed to anything "medical," only basic biology and chemistry stuff. Out there, if they were shot or otherwise wounded, I could help, but if they were sick, then I was completely useless.

Also, I had to adapt to basic lifestyle changes. To go for days without some sort of bath was the norm out there, while here it is regarded as disgusting.

Sleeping in the sand was common, and to be able to sleep on a cot was considered a luxury. Voiding/defecating was pretty much where you felt like it, as long as the smell didn't blow downwind of the vehicle. Defecating without the luxury of a toilet or anything to sit on or even lean on is quite an experience. Dig a hole and try it someday if you think it is easy.

For me, there were very little support mechanisms. Whatever I experienced, I experienced alone. I was the only one from my reserve unit that was assignment to that unit. As a matter of fact, they weren't expecting me when I arrived. I was a complete surprise to them, and of course, they had not made such provisions as finding for me a place to sleep or even a vehicle to ride in. The regulars out there really didn't like me. I was a stranger. I didn't know a damn thing, and I had a lot of luggage. Those soldiers around my own age already had established clicks, of which I was not invited. By the first of April, there was a rumor that I was from the Central Intelligence Division, or CID. They were supposedly known to do things like drop their people off in a unit at awkward times to see if they do anything illegal like keep foreign weapons. Oddly enough, I had not even heard of the Central Intelligence Division until I was accused of being in it!

Needless to say, I was pretty much ostracized from that group. The older soldiers did not believe it, but they too had their clicks. They shared different interests than I did, and so I really did not connect with any of them. Essentially, I was alone.

It's a very odd feeling to be thrown into a situation in which literally everything is different. The climate was different, the people, the plants, the animals, everything. Even the stars seemed akilter somehow. They were definitely brighter out there, since the sky was so clear (when the oil smoke didn't blow over us). I remember one particular clear night where a few of us were sitting around just admiring the stars at night. That night was very quiet, at least until a heated argument broke out as to the exact location of the Big Dipper. I had borrowed a pair of binoculars that one of the men had found in a headquarters building in Safwan and was looking at the moon. The sky was so clear that I could actually get a good look at the moon's craters. That's quite different from Muncie's nights, where to be able to even see the moon at night is almost a miracle.

I guess perhaps the clear sky and the dry air were the only things that I really liked out there. I really liked the dry air. Living in the Ohio Valley all my life, I could not believe it when my sinuses cleared up for the first time. However, that's not worth the scorpions, the heat, the sand, and the flies.

The only ties I had to the life that I left were the things I had brought with me. These included a few pictures, everything that was in my wallet, a few civilian clothes, and the headphones and cassette tapes that I bought in Jackson the day before I shipped out. I had no way of contacting friends and family back home for over a month after I got there. I did not have an address to give to them so that they could write me until after the ground war was over. It took about a week after the offensive was over before mail started filtering through to us. Of course, I would not get any of it for a long time. From the time that I sent out a letter until the time that someone received it here at the States was about three to four weeks. It only took eight days to receive a letter, so that was over a month from the time that I sent a letter until I received one. The first contact that I had with anyone from home was on March 18, the first time that I got to use the phone. It was not for another week or so after that before I got my first letter.

Things were so different over there for me that after a while I had trouble remembering what life was like at home. It all seemed like some movie that I saw a long time ago, like none of it was reality. Perhaps this was a way that I could cope with the utter strangeness of it all. I don't know. I would dream of the States, and it was not my life. It was something else that I may or may not have experienced once. I was isolated there, and I had no contact with the "real" world. After a while, I stopped dreaming of home.

That may sound a little farfetched, but it's the truth. Not everyone experienced the same things over there, nor reacted the same way to the war, and I'm sure that no one experienced what I did. The diary only tells what I saw. It doesn't tell what I felt. It doesn't tell about the constant badgering that I received out there from certain members of that unit, because I was a reservist, because I was new. It doesn't fully describe the knot in my stomach every time an explosion would rattle our track. It also doesn't describe the annoyance (frustration?) that I would feel when I would wake up and realize that I was still there, and still alone.

When I returned, I suffered from post-traumatic stress disorder, or PTSD. For about four months after returning to the Midwest from the desert, I suffered from depression, anxiety, weight gain, restlessness, and I was easily startled, especially when I heard sounds that reminded me of explosions or gunfire. Anxiety attacks were the normal rather than the unusual. One doesn't have to be in a war, however, to experience PTSD. It can be experienced by anyone who has had some sort of traumatic experience; the military just put a name to it. For example, if someone was in a car accident and was having problem coping with it—having nightmares or anxiety attacks whenever they ride in a car—it's essentially the same thing.

Here again, I was to go through another transition. One would think that the return trip would be easier, and yet in reality it is a hundred times harder. Why was the return trip so difficult? That is a question that I am still asking myself. I think it is because I expected life to return to "normal" when I came home. Perhaps I thought that the world that I left would be the same one that I was returning to. However, that was not the case. I was not the same person when I returned, nor were they the same people that I left. Everyone was a stranger, and it took time to get reacquainted. Also, not only were the people different, the world in general was not the same one that I left. Life continued while I was gone, and I missed part of it. Even now, someone will make a reference to something that happened during that time, and I have to remind him or her that I wasn't here then. The phase around my house is "it happened when you were gone," like I blinked into nonexistence for three months or something.

Another symptom of PTSD is the constant reliving of the experience. I had a very hard time trying not to think about the desert. Dreams of the war were common, which made it even harder to try to find this life when I was still living the other one. Eventually, though, they faded away, and now I only dream about it once in a great while.

How did I cope once I returned? Oddly enough, I don't think I really did. I think that I just kept at it long enough, and things worked themselves out. There was not much that I could really do; I just survived until I could get a handle on things. I think that I was very fortunate to get home in time for summer vacation. I spent the entire summer thinking. I thought about what I had just gone through and what I was going to do now that it was over.

Once school started that fall, I was still a little wobbly about some things, like my relationship with my girlfriend, and definitely touchy whenever someone mentioned the war, especially during drill weekends. Whenever a group of desert vets got together, the topic invariable would turn to the war. It still happens, two years later; it seems like each one tries to outdo the others in his or her stories, whether it be of fun times spent in Kuwait City or the hardships endured in the desert. Personally, whenever they start mentioning the desert, I just feel sick. I would prefer to get on with my life and let the experience fade into hazy memories where they belong.

The experience wasn't completely a negative one, though. I did bring home some very neat souvenirs. I have two Iraqi gas masks, an Iraqi flag that I found in a headquarters building in Safwan, quite a few of those pamphlets that we dropped on the Iraqis telling than to surrender, a canteen, a complete Iraqi uniform (again from the headquarters building), and an Iraqi license plate that I took off of a burned-out car (an American car, no less) that was in the road.

Also, I don't think I have ever been as emotionally touched as when I shook hands with my father when I came home, and I saw the pride in his eyes. At that moment, I probably felt closer to him than I ever have in my life.

The experience has definitely altered me. I think that now I have a greater awareness and definition of myself. While I was out there, I had plenty of time to analyze my life, and myself. I learned a lot about myself out there. I know myself, and that is something that a lot of us will never really achieve.

During those first few days, I did not know whether or nor I was going to live or die any time soon. That is a disturbing thing to think about. Also disturbing is why I was out there in the first place. Was it for democracy or for national security? Hell no, I was there to protect our oil interests, pure and simple. I was out there risking my life so that we could keep gas prices down. At the time, I thought that my uniform should have had Property of OPEC rather than US Army. What a cause I was willing to die for!

I'm sure that we all think about death every once in a while—I know I have—but to really be confronted with it is something else entirely. To actually wonder if this is going to be the last day on earth is frightening. But I did gain something from the experience. I confronted my own morality, and I have come to terms with it. I became comfortable with the idea that I am mortal. I will eventually die like the rest of us. How would I spend the day if I knew that it was the last day of my life? I wouldn't change a thing. What I am doing now is what I would want to be doing if I were to die tomorrow (except perhaps not sit here all day typing). I am doing what I want to do.

I'm also much more patient and tolerant now than I was before I left. There are very little things now that upset me. Why? Probably because I can now look at them in perspective. The trials and tribulations that we all face each and every day are nothing compared to the trials and tribulations that I faced in the desert.

Another big change for me is my greater appreciation of nature. The natural world is something that we miss here in America because we live in an antiseptic, sequestered life as far away from nature as we can possibly get. We wake up in a climate-controlled house that is more or less animal free, we get in a car that is the same, and we usually work in a place that is not nature. Even when we "go out to nature," it really isn't natural, but a facsimile of it. State parks and forests, provided that we go to them at all, have been altered for our recreation enjoyment. There are roads leading directly to a camping spot where we pitch a tent to keep out of the elements; we even bring with us most of the comforts of home, half of which we don't really need. All we essentially do is move the house to a different location for a few days. Most places have bathroom facilities at our fingertips, and God forbid if there's no toilet paper!

We rush too much in America. Everything is on a timetable. We even have to plan when to relax—and dare not relax any longer than that or we will be late for something. We're also bombarded with too much external stimuli. How can we even take time out with so much floating past us, demanding our attention? When I was in the desert, the land and the people had remained essentially unchanged for centuries. Sure, some of the Bedouins drove Mitsubishi trucks instead of rode camels, but some of them did have camel herds. Out there, there was no real timetable. Most of the time here, we rush and don't even realize it. Out there, all the days were the same, differing only with the passing seasons. Those people did not rush, because there was no reason to.

The sheer enormity of nature out there was overwhelming. As far as the eye could see—which was pretty damn far, because it was completely flat out there, and there was no trees to create an artificial horizon—was nothing but nature, nothing man-made at all. That's quite a change from Indiana. I spent the greater portion of two months surrounded by nature. I lived in it. It was actually very beautiful (as long as we weren't in a part of the country where the actual fighting took place).

On the down side, though, were there any long-term problems caused form the war? That's something that I'm still thinking about and something that I may never have an answer to. The biggest concern that I have is whether or not the smoke form the oil fires affected me in a way that might not turn up for another ten years or so. Also, I know that even now I cannot donate blood until 1994 because I had to take malaria tablets and other, equally nasty stuff. I guess the jury's still out on this, and I won't know unless something happens. I can guess that I didn't contract some exotic parasite, because something like that would have been apparent by now, I hope.

There are two nagging questions that I still ask myself. One is whether in general, this experience was a good one or a bad one. I think that it had both qualities. On the short term, the experience itself was very unpleasant, and the initial homecoming not much better. However, as I get further and further in time from the actual event, I increasingly feel that there are some things that I gained from this experience. I am a much stronger person for having done what I did, and I am, in a way, happier because I did it. I really have little doubt in my mind as to what I want to do with the rest of my life, and that allows me to be more focused in what I do. I can concentrate on what I am doing without having that nagging little voice whispering in my ear, asking me if I am really happy doing this.

The second question is, if I had to do this again, would I have volunteered to go? That's a good one. When I initially made the decision, I was really thinking about the men with wives and children that they would have to leave. I really don't know what I would do if I had to decide again. I do know, however, that I don't regret the decision. At the time, I thought that it was the correct one to make.

And so life goes on.

Twenty-two years later, I still have occasional nightmares. I probably always will. I do not wish to feel self-important by running off to watch as the coroner scrapes some guy off the pavement. I want to prevent that. I wish to help others when I can and by all means not be the cause of it. Paraprofessionals know enough to be good at what they do, but they cannot see the whole picture. For a radiology tech, once the picture is shot, then they're responsibility is over. Yet they have the "authority" to dictate the pace and direction of patient care. For an EMT the "run" is over when the patient is dropped off in the ER. That's when my job starts, and that patient is my "baby" until they either find another doctor or die. I have almost four thousand "children" that I take care of and am responsible for. I am not proud of what I do; I am in awe of it.

# Shift Mentality

Unfortunately shift mentality is pretty prevalent in the health care field, especially among nursing and other allied health professions. I haven't seen any studies that show that it's a detriment to patient care, but as a physician trying to take care of someone, it sure is a pain in the ass. [43]

I define shift mentality simply as clocking in and out as specific times according to a schedule. I understand that not everyone is on salary or available twenty-four hours a day like I am. Almost the entire industrialized world operates on a shift schedule. I get that. As an ER tech and a CNA, I was all about shift work. I also understand that with the exception of bitching about disrupted sleep, there are no detrimental effects of working exclusively nights to either the workers or their patients. Here's a scenario, however, in which shift mentality bites me in the ass:

Nurse from the nursing home calls me at 8:00 p.m. on Friday night: "Doctor, Mr. Smithers looks really bad. His legs are swollen, he's not breathing well, and he is complaining of severe chest pain."

Me: "Hmm, sounds serious. Probably need to send him to the emergency room for evaluation."

ER doc six hours later: "Hey, why's Smithers here? He looks better than he normally does. I've looked and can't find anything. His first set of labs, ekg, and chest X-rays are normal."

Me: "Dunno, nurse said he looked like hell. Couldn't breathe, low oxygen saturation, chest pain."

ER doc: "Well, if he looked that bad, then I recommend we at least admit him for observation to rule out a small heart attack."

Me (groaning): "Okay, tuck him in, and I'll see him in the morning."

And so he gets admitted. I wander in on Saturday morning to find that he looks better than I have seen him recently. He has no complaints, and his workup is normal. I pat him on the head and send him home.

Here's my theory:

Nurse shows up at the nursing home after being off for four days. She has three glorious twelve-hour shifts to look forward to this weekend, and as soon as she's done, she is going on a trip to Gatlinburg with her new boyfriend. She doesn't know which hall she has to take care of until she gets there, and she's in no mood to put up with anyone's shit tonight. She prays it's not the 300 hall, because that sonofabitch Smithers is on that hall.

Well, wouldn't you know it? She gets the 300 hall. Smithers is hitting the call light every ten minutes complaining about something, and she can't get any of her other work done. If she only had a sleeping pill to give him her life would be much easier. Unfortunately that's not an option.

Smithers decides he's gonna choke on his drink at dinner. He's supposed to be on thickened liquids, because he tends to choke on anything else. He decided last week that he wasn't going to drink that crap and signed a waiver stating that he takes full responsibility if he doesn't follow the recommendations of the speech therapist. I've okayed it, because he's a big boy and not demented (although mean as hell) and can make his own health care decisions. I've explained to him in excruciating detail that he will likely choke on something, and it will go into his lungs. He will subsequently get aspiration pneumonia and likely die from this. He is fully aware and okay with this. I'm not going to babysit him. If he wants to drink soda and die, he for the time being still has that right as an American citizen. The government hasn't taken that decision away from him yet.

Well that's what happens tonight. Nurse Gatlinburg now has to get up from charting to fix him, because he's turning blue. She slaps a pulse oximeter on him and checks his oxygen saturations. Fortunately for her his oxygen saturations are in the low 80s, which is well below the 92 percent or above we would like him to live at. His chest hurts, because he's been coughing for the past few minutes. His legs are swollen, because he won't take his water pill. It makes him have to pee all day, and he doesn't like that, so he won't take it. So now Nurse Gatlinburg steps back and looks at him. He is having low oxygen saturations, he has complained of chest pain, and he is having leg swelling. Hmm, must be time to call the doctor. After all, we need to let him know what is going on. She wouldn't want to be held responsible for not calling the doctor. Nurses do have licenses that they must protect, just like physicians. Okay, so she calls me. I can't see him through the phone obviously, and based on what was told to me, he needs to see someone. Off to the ER.

So the nurse calls the ambulance to take him to the ER. The EMTs arrive with lights and sirens. (It's fun to blow through stoplights. Been there, done that.) By the time they arrive, he is pretty much back to baseline. His oxygen is in the mid 90 percent, he has stopped coughing, but he is annoyed because NCIS is about to start, and he wants to watch television. The EMTs package him up anyway (doctor's orders after all), and they swing by the ER just long enough to drop him and his paperwork off. Their shift is over in about forty-five minutes by now, and they have to get back to the garage and finish some paperwork. They don't stick around long enough to give a report to the ER physician, who is about two hours behind at this point.

By the time the ER doc gets to see Mr. Smithers, it's somewhere around 11:00 p.m. He does the usual and customary workup based on the scant information that he has from the EMT run sheet. The nursing note from the home only states, "Spoke to physician, pt to ER for evaluation." The patient has no complaints at this point and doesn't know why he is even there. It's now somewhere between two and three in the morning. He calls me; we chat. The worst thing we could do is send him back to the nursing home if he did indeed have a small heart attack. That's where lawsuits come from. Smithers wants everything done to him up to and including chest compressions and being placed on a ventilator. He has an estranged son living in Arizona who apparently has some unresolved guilt issues because he likes to call and threaten legal action if "everything isn't done" but doesn't quite care enough to actually fly out here and visit.

Unfortunately it might be from six to eighteen hours before we can answer the heart attack question with any certainty. The condition we are concerned about is called subendocardial myocardial infarction (that's fancy Latin for small heart attack). Smithers therefore gets admitted, and Nurse Gatlinburg doesn't have to deal with him this shift.

I wish this was the exception to the rule, but I can expect some variation of this almost every weekend. One Saturday I was rounding on my nursing home patients after working in the office for the morning. I had popped in to see a couple of people whom I was past due to see. One of them was a sweet old lady. No issues or problems with her with the exception of some arthritis, which hadn't been bothering her recently. When I saw her she was sitting comfortably up in her chair eating lunch and watching television. She was smiling and comfortable. She had no complaints, and her exam was unchanged from the previous two-dozen exams I had given her. I had just left the parking lot of the nursing home when I get a call from the nurse stating that Grandma Sweetness was in excruciating pain and needed to be transferred to the ER for evaluation. Okay, I understand that people sometimes go bad faster than potato salad in July, but this didn't seem right. I turned around and wandered back in to see her still sitting in her chair where I had left her, still smiling.

Another effect of shift work that I see is that there is lack of continuity. Even when everyone is competent and means well, it takes a little while to learn each patient. Yes, unlike the nursing profession, I use the term patient, not client. I am their physician; therefore, they are my patients. They are not clients—I am not a lawyer or prostitute, nor do I work for an advertising agency.

If there were some consistency in regards to which nurse gets which patients from one day to the next, it might help. Patients who have been in the hospital for a while might not have the same nurse twice, which seems to me makes continuity of care difficult. My experience is this varies widely from institution to institution.

Don't ever try to get anything done at 6:00 a.m. or 6:00 p.m.—ironically the two best times for me to see patients at the hospital. Shift change is somewhere around 7:00. Starting at 6:00 no one wants to do anything. A transfer from the ER would require that the floor nurse do the proper assessments and mountain of paperwork required before she goes home. I certainly understand the hesitancy to want to stay even longer after a twelve-hour shift. It just makes it difficult to get anything done then. I've had patients sit in the ER for hours longer than they needed simply because the admission orders were written around shift change. I've also argued as early as last weekend with the ER physician who was reluctant to transfer someone to a larger hospital that could more properly care for a patient because it was too close to shift change. Again, shift mentality is a pain in the ass.

# Research

I will be the first to tell you that I am no mathematician or researcher, nor do I pretend to be. However, the blatant misuse or abuse of research and statistics appalls me. I would like to think that those doing research in medicine would at least try to be objective or at least truthful. Unfortunately, that is not the case. I would also like to think that the media would use a little more common sense when reporting "breakthrough" medical studies, but since that kind of thing makes for a great story on a slow news day, I guess that will never happen.

The classic example of an abomination that was called research is a study done by Andrew Wakefield. In 1998 he published a paper that showed a link between the Measles, Mumps, and Rubella (MMR) vaccine and autism. It was subsequently proved that he intentionally manipulated his research data.[44]

Thankfully the study had been retracted, and it appears that he can now no longer practice medicine, but unfortunately the damage has already been done. My personal experience is that his original paper in 1998 had a profound effect on the psyche of the Americans and their views of immunizations. I cannot count the number of parents in my office that refused immunizations to their children due this paper. This also has international implications affecting not just in my little corner of America. Before publication of Wakefield's findings, the inoculation rate for MMR in the UK was 92 percent; after publication, the rate dropped to below 80 percent. In 1998, there were 56 measles cases in the UK; by 2008, there were 1348 cases, with two confirmed deaths.[45]

We give immunizations for a reason. That is, to prevent diseases that have in the past caused significant morbidity and mortality for the population as a whole. Unfortunately, we now live in a time when we do not know what it is like to live with smallpox, measles, or polio as examples, and this leads to complacency among parents. Take a study such as the one Wakefield published, and that gives people greater reason to not immunize their children. For example, from 1998 to 2003 there has been a 23 percent increase in hospitalization rates for children with pertussis.[46] In 2010 there were about 27,550 cases of whooping cough in the United States, one of the highest numbers in over fifty years.[47] One of the foundations of public health is immunization against disease. Despite strong recommendations by the Centers for Disease Control and Prevention, this most basic tenant also seems to be forgotten or ignored by the very government that is supposed to protect us.

The Vaccine for Children (VFC) program is a federal program that provides eligible children all recommended vaccines at no cost.[48] You may, however, be charged a small processing fee. The federal government pays for the vaccines, and doctors and clinics agree to give the vaccines to children who qualify. That sounds like a great idea. But who, you ask, does this cover? Can I get my child his mandatory immunizations? To answer those questions the CDC provides us with a brochure. Let's see what it means to be eligible:

> Children from birth through 18 years of age can receive vaccines through the VFC program if they are at least one of the following: eligible for Medicaid, without health insurance, American Indian or Alaska Native, or under-insured. If you have health insurance that doesn't cover

vaccines, your child is eligible. However, you will have to go to a federally qualified health center or a rural health clinic for your VFC vaccinations. Call your local or state health department immunization program for a center nearest you.

Sounds decent maybe, except in my corner of the world there are no federally qualified health centers or rural health clinics within, well, anywhere.

So I guess you must go to your private physician's office for immunizations, except your doctor doesn't carry them. Immunization reimbursement from insurance carriers is typically at or less than the cost of the immunization itself, not taking into account the cost for storage and staff time. Immunizations do expire. My office once lost a significant amount of money, in the thousands of dollars, simply by miscalculating the number of influenza immunizations needed. That was an expensive lesson. The following year we did not order as many. Once those we ordered were gone, we no longer offered the immunization for the rest of the season. Being financially solvent took precedence over public health. That is tragic. Unfortunately the options were that or potentially lose money. A physician in bankruptcy does no one any good at all. Once again, the cost of practicing medicine is more than the return. Go get the oil changed on your car, then not only refuse to pay the mechanic, ask him for ten bucks. It's the same.

If you do have insurance, it's still questionable whether you can get the shots even if you can find someone who carries them. Some insurance carriers cover immunizations without cost to the patient, some will charge it toward the deductible, and some do not cover at all. A single vaccine, (such as the shingles vaccine) can cost upward of three hundred dollars, and most vaccines are in series of two or more.

In my office we understand that the need for public health sometimes outweighs the potential financial risk. After all, we went into medicine to help people. We do offer all childhood immunizations required by the state and those common immunizations that are necessary to provide comprehensive population-based medical care. We sometimes break even, and sometimes we do not.

Research of the blatantly obvious is also what I call "no kidding, Sherlock" research. Okay, change out kidding for a more explicit euphemism. I'm not sure if there's a Latin phrase for that. (It would be cool if there was—everything in medicine should have a Latin phrase attached to it.) I don't know if it upsets me more because it's ridiculous; it's what the media seems to like to latch on to, or because people talk about it like it's such a medical breakthrough. Maybe it's because I didn't think of getting it published first (like I have time to do that). My favorite examples that epitomize this are two classics: "Most accidents happen at home" and, "Most car accidents occur within a few miles of home." I would like to use these examples as a good foundation for thinking about research.

Let's think about these two for a moment. Where are we most likely to do stupid stuff? At work where we can get fired or in our backyards when no one is looking? Where do we spend roughly two-thirds of our time? (Hopefully you're not at work.) Where are we placed in situations where we can be exposed to mind or coordination-altering substances (legal or otherwise) and be within arm's reach of sharp, explosive, elevated, or otherwise dangerous objects? Never mind the basics such as the icy sidewalk or the loose carpet. (Where's the chainsaw? Ahh, there it is right next to my rickety old ladder. Now, where's my gas can? Hold my beer and watch this...) Where do you most of your driving? Where do you do most of your driving while eating a cheeseburger, texting on the phone, and trying to reach in the back seat and pick up that soda your kid just spilled all over the carpet of your new car on the way to the soccer practice that you are already ten minutes late? If you answered home/near home then you are well on your way to being a researcher. This isn't rocket science.

Of course, I didn't read either studies if in fact they exist. Who has time for that? Like most of you, I learn about "medical breakthroughs" from the media outlets, which don't go into any details. Perhaps these studies went into more detail. Perhaps they controlled for accidents per minute at home versus accidents per minute not at home rather than total accidents, or accidents per activity for that matter. For example, do more loggers get hurt cutting wood at home or cutting wood at work? Maybe they corrected for the fact that most of us rarely take roadtrips, and adjusted for this by comparing the ratios of accidents per hours driven near home versus accidents per hours driven away from home rather than comparing the absolute numbers. Maybe these are just urban myths that we perpetuate. I don't know, but you've probably heard about them just as I have.

Hell, let me throw some statistics at you that some of you may find mind-blowing: Most people in the United States sleep in a bed. More breakfast is eaten in the morning than any other time of day. People on blood thinners tend to bleed more than people not on blood thinners. People who take stimulants will feel better for a short time than those who don't. The sun is seen more often during the day. I could go on, but I think the point is obvious. Unfortunately, some of those statements are actual research that I have seen on the national news.

The next is misleading research. Just because something sounds wonderful in a "study" doesn't make it the panacea for all your problems. Coffee and alcohol are two substances that as of late seem to be making the rounds. If I took at face value what I hear about these two substances, I could live forever on beer and coffee. Between the two of them they have been shown to enhance cognitive function, improve mood, protect against heart disease, and decrease the risk of type 2 diabetes and stroke if taken in moderation.[49,50] That sounds wonderful. Where do I sign up? However, that is not the entire picture. Adverse effects can include such things as hypertension (which actually increases risk for heart disease and stroke), gastritis (inflammation of the stomach lining, which can lead to bleeding ulcers, which one would think would tend to bleed more if you are on blood thinners; although I haven't seen a study supporting that idea), heart arrhythmias, cirrhosis of the liver, anxiety, depression, and making poor social decisions at 2:00 a.m.[51]

Let me talk about statistics for a minute. Statistics can be manipulated in all sorts of ways to make whatever point you want, and this is yet another way in which the science of medicine gets distorted. In my practice, I deal with risk on a daily basis. I live and breathe risk, and almost everything I do involves the probability of something or other happening or not happening to someone. Sometimes that's me trying to reduce my risk of getting sued, and sometimes it's me trying to reduce the risk of your untimely death, but either way it involves risk.

Generally speaking, risk is described three ways. In other words, depending on the situation we can make something sound really horrible or really good depending what point is trying to be made. To better understand how this works, let's discuss probability or likelihood. For example, the likelihood of a woman in the United States developing breast cancer in her lifetime is roughly 12 percent or one in eight.[52] So, depending on the point you are trying to make, that can sound horrible or not so bad. If I am trying to instill fear in you so that you'll run around wearing pink and donating to causes, I'll tell you that you have a one in eight chance of developing breast cancer in your lifetime. If I am trying to console you then I will tell you that you have an 88 percent chance of not developing breast cancer in your lifetime. So depending on your politics, this can be described either way.

Unfortunately for breast cancer, this is still a pretty high number, and maybe we all need to be out trying to save the ta tas. Personally I look silly in pink, but whatever. For other diseases, however, the numbers are much lower, and the description of risk becomes more interesting. For example, using some nifty on-line calculator that I found, I can plug in my medical information (which apparently almost anyone can get without my consent or knowledge), and it tells me that my risk for a heart attack within the next ten years is roughly 1 percent.[53] That means that one in one hundred people with my risk factors will have a heart attack. Okay, so what does this have to do with anything? We are now back to the three ways that risk is described.

Let's continue discussing the real-life example of my risk for a heart attack over the next ten years. If I take a medicine or do something, like heaven forbid eat better and exercise, I might be able to get that risk to less than 1 percent. Or, conversely, if I do something bad, like grow old and wind up on Medicare, my risk could go higher than 1 percent. If I decrease my risk of a heart attack from 1 percent to 0.7 percent, then I have demonstrated what is called an absolute risk reduction. That is, my risk has gone down that much. That doesn't sound very impressive given the fact that the likelihood of my having a heart attack wasn't all that high to begin with.

However, another way to describe this is by using a trick called relative risk reduction. In relative risk reduction terms, I have now reduced my risk for a heart attack by 30 percent. That sounds much more impressive, especially if I am trying to sell you something. The other way this is used is as a scare tactic. If my risk of some horrible side effect is 1 percent, and by taking this medication it now becomes 2 percent, I have doubled my risk of having this horrible and potentially life threatening side effect. Lawyers love this one. If you took medication X, then you are twice as likely to develop side effect Y. Call me, and I'll be more than happy to file a class action lawsuit...

The other way risk is described is something called number needed to treat. If I have a medication that reduces your risk of developing some badness, such as a heart attack, by 1 percent, then I have to treat one hundred patients before I see the benefits of using this medication on one person. To be perfectly honest, I don't know how this last description of risk is useful in any practical sense in my private practice. Either a medication is FDA approved and recommended to treat a particular condition, or it isn't. I don't count the number of times I have prescribed a certain medication so I can keep tabs on the numbers I have treated and therefore statistics on how many people I have "saved," so it seems like a silly statistic in my book. I've seen some nerdy types get all worked up about this for some reason, so I'll mention it for completeness' sake. I suppose I could see it being used as a benchmark by the government or insurance companies to determine whether a treatment is "worth" the financial cost.

In my office I often talk about the lottery. It's an example everyone is familiar with.

Patient: "Doctor, I don't want to take this medicine. I saw on TV that it doubles my risk for congestive heart failure [or other equally nasty problem]."

Me: "Let's talk about risk. There are two kinds of risk, what I call absolute risk and relative risk. Have you ever played the lottery?"

Patient: "Sure."

Me: "Okay, so you know that the odds of you winning the state lottery are somewhere around one in twelve million. We both agree that those are pretty crappy odds, right?" [I usually don't swear in the exam room. Grandma gets upset.]

Patient: "Yes."

Me: "Now, if I buy another lottery ticket, my odds are two in twelve million. That's still pretty lousy odds, right?"

Patient: "Ah, yes."

Me: "However, if I were trying to influence you, I would tell you that your odds of winning the lottery have just doubled."

Patient: "Yes, but those are still pretty low odds."

Me: "Good, you understand. Now we can talk about if you want to stop this medicine, but we also need to talk about the risk of something bad happening to you if you don't take this medicine or one like it." At that point the discussion becomes more reasonable.

Hindsight is twenty-twenty, or the retrospective study. Generally speaking, I don't have an issue with retrospective studies, but when they are used to create treatment recommendations, it gets rather problematic. My favorite example of this is bronchitis.

Any cursory browse through the Internet will show you that the "experts" say that antibiotics are not indicated for the treatment of acute bronchitis. The reason being is that the vast majorities of cases are viral in nature and are self-limiting. Therefore antibiotics are useless and should not be used. Okay. I understand that, but let's look at this a little closer.

Signs and symptoms of acute viral bronchitis can include: cough, sputum production, malaise, low-grade elevation in temperature, headache, muscle aches, shortness of breath, chest pain, and wheezing. The physical exam can be from normal to wheezing to respiratory distress.[54]

Pneumonia, which is an infection (usually bacterial) in the lungs, is almost always treated with antibiotics and can be life threatening in certain circumstances.

Signs and symptoms of pneumonia can include: cough, sputum production, malaise, low-grade elevation in temperature, headache, muscle aches, shortness of breath, chest pain, and wheezing. The physical exam can be from normal to wheezing to respiratory distress.[55]

So you can see the dilemma. When someone walks in the exam room, and keeping everything else equal, it is difficult to impossible to tell one from the other. Even with X-rays and labs, they can look the same. Patients often don't wait the obligatory seven to ten days before they wander in to see me. Two to four days is more like the average in my corner of the world. Now last I checked I don't have a crystal ball. I can't tell you with any certainty whether what you are presenting to me with is just a viral bronchitis or an early pneumonia. My internal lawyer will tell me to treat the worst-case scenario. Congratulations, you just got an antibiotic. 80 percent of all cases of bronchitis get antibiotics.[56] Is there any wonder?

What burns my biscuit though is when I am held responsible from a retrospective standpoint. In this case, I am held responsible for prescribing antibiotics for what eventually turned out to be a viral bronchitis. Okay, that's not too bad. I can deal with that until insurance companies start reducing my payments for treatment or giving me a bad "score" based on clinical outcomes, such as the treatment of viral bronchitis with antibiotics. I also don't appreciate, but in a much bigger way, when I elect not to give someone antibiotics and they eventually end up getting pneumonia. That starts to smell a lot like malpractice depending on the ultimate outcome of the patient and the laws in your particular state. If someone dies three days after they see me and I treat them for "bronchitis" with a little chicken soup and some TLC, the family of the deceased get a little snippy. Been there, got that T-shirt, thanks. I will over treat every time.

My other favorite statistical myth is that most health care dollars are spent in the last six months of life. I was going to use this as an example of the retrospective study, but it appears that it's just an incorrect statement. Unfortunately, I've heard politicians use this as a starting place to discuss limiting certain treatments in the elderly. Without going into too much politics, that just seems to me to be a dangerous place to be. Here in America, we pride ourselves in being free and choosing our own destinies. Should the government decide who gets what treatment? By limiting the payment of such services, Uncle Sam has de facto made the decision of what medical treatment is "best" for us, just like insurance companies already do now. If you don't believe me, try getting a PET scan "just because."

On average only 10 percent of someone's total medical expenditures are spent in the last six months of life. However, if one would look at this differently, approximately 27 percent of Medicare dollars are spent in the last year of life.[57] That makes sense given Medicare's demographic. It's not designed for the young and healthy last I checked. However, almost 50 percent (48.6 percent actually) of all health care dollars are spent in those sixty-five years and older. I suppose if one would prefer to save money, then starting with the 1976 movie Logan's Run would be a good place to begin.[58] You just turned 30? Happy birthday. Time for you to get vaporized. I know there has been some debate regarding how Medicare dollars are spent and whether this money is better spent somewhere else. I guess if my crystal ball was working and I knew that the person I was treating was going to die in six months, I could change my treatment perhaps to save Uncle Sam a few bucks. It's easy to go back and say, "Gee, doctor, everything you did was futile. You should have stopped trying months ago".

Unfortunately, last I checked I was morally and legally obligated to prevent and treat disease, and anything less is malpractice. Again, I do not know the time or the place, and it is not my decision to make. I will save that one for someone else. The hard discussions about end-of-life planning in theory should have taken place before we have gotten to this point. In many cases, however, despite our best efforts, we are now there without any clear guidance, and the treatment decisions must be made between me and the patient or the patient's family—if the patient is unable at that time. From experience, the decision to withhold treatment or do less than "everything possible" is a difficult one to make.

Cum hoc ergo propter hoc (Latin for "with this, therefore because of this") is a logical fallacy that can be seen in medical research.[59] It is also called "correlation proves causation."

It is epitomized in the classic example of ice cream and crime. The argument is this: It has been shown that as ice cream sales increase, so does the crime rate. Therefore, ice cream must lead to crime. In this particular argument, it does not take into account that both an increase in ice cream sales and an increase in crime rates both occur during the summer months. Crime rates increase during the summer for numerous other reasons, not because ice cream was sold.

Another, more familiar example that had real world implications was the correlation between hormone replacement in women and the risk of heart disease. The argument there was women who took hormone replacement after menopause had a lower risk of heart disease. It took further research to show that this was a logical fallacy; those taking hormone replacements had other variables, such as better diet and exercise programs, that reduced their risk of having heart disease.[60]

Unfortunately, I'm still undoing that one. I spent the first eight years of medical practicing pimping out estrogen to the postmenopausal, and now I've spent at least an equal amount trying to undo that. I better hurry before some hold out still on hormone replacement has a heart attack. I've seen the commercials on television. Lawyers are out there looking. Eighty-seven percent rate of malpractice suit...

The point is, think about what you hear before taking it at face value. Understand that doctors base their recommendations and practice methods on the best information they have at that time. If you have any questions, please ask your doctor before you make up your mind about something based on a "study" you heard about on the nightly news.

# The Almighty Health Care Dollar

Let's sit down and have a beer for this section; we're both going to need it. If you prefer to not have a beer, then have a beverage of your choice; although alcohol in moderation has shown to have health benefits. What exactly is this health care dollar? Very simply, it is the money that is spent in the United States for any aspect of health care.[61] This is a contentious topic, which is debated incessantly both in the general public as well as on Capitol Hill. I won't pretend to understand it all, but I do understand it where it affects us, at the individual level. After all, at the end of the day either we can afford to go to the doctor or we can't.

Let me explain it in its most simple form. I will start with beer. Besides working and co-parenting my children, my other love is brewing beer. I suppose it might be making rum, but since we have laws in place regarding distillation that make home distillation impractical if not illegal in many states, I'll stick to beer. Not that I get to drink much of it given my schedule, but it's the process of creating that I enjoy. Besides, it's a good use of my biology degree.

Beer brewing, like health care, can be as simple or as complicated as you want it to be. At its most basic form brewing beer, or raising bread if you prefer, requires only two things: yeast and yeast food. In the health care model, I will be the yeast. I will take the food (a patient) and do something to him or her. Remember, the practice of medicine in its most basic form is the evaluation and treatment of a patient by a physician. In brewing, fermentation is the conversion of sugar (food) into alcohol (a waste product) by yeast. So far so good?

Beyond this step beer brewing gets very complicated very quickly.[62] Beers are classified into different types by the yeast used. Lager yeast differs from ale yeast. Hops (a type of vine) are added for flavor as well as preservation. There is what seems like an infinite variety of hops, each grown for specific flavor, aroma, or bitterness. Brewing times and fermentation temperatures vary. Equipment can range from a simple five-gallon plastic bucket to a multi-million dollar brewery. Terminology becomes very complex very quickly. Malt, hops, wort, sparging, mashing, trub, and carboy are common terms. Measuring conventions include specific gravity, IBUs, AAUs, and Lovibond color scales. We must be careful not to cause disruption of the fermentation process by environmental contaminants such as natural yeast and bacteria, so there must be a process for preventing this. In very short order the forest is lost for the trees, as they say. One is soon drowning in too much information, and the basics are forgotten.

In medicine it is the same problem. There are different types of doctors. Are you a lager or ale, an osteopath or allopath? What variety of hop are you, a cardiologist or pediatrician? Where do you do your best work, clinic or hospital, a five-gallon plastic bucket at home or a five hundred-gallon copper fermenter in a professional brewery? What other environmental factors are influencing the fermentation process? Are the wild yeast of chiropractors, homeopathic practitioners, or other practitioners or paraprofessionals muddying the waters and contaminating the substrate, the patient?

Medical terminology is classically complex. I am going to digress for a moment and talk about medical terminology. From a physician's practical standpoint, medical terminology is a necessary evil. Just like all aspects of medicine, it is also being eroded. Unfortunately, terminology was created and is utilized for a reason. One compliment that I receive from my patients consistently is my ability to speak to them in a language that they understand. My response is invariably that I don't know any other way to speak to them. I simply convert what I know into words that I have always used. I save the Latin for the chart. Medical terminology is not to make medicine occult and elitist. It is used to specifically convey a very large amount of information in a very concise format, similar to a computer zip file today. There are also two aspects to medical language that must be considered: terminology and abbreviations. Take this example of an order that I might write to a nurse or on a prescription:

Apply i gtt ou qd to bid et hs prn
Or these physical examination findings:

Gen: NAD.

Heent: NCAT, PERRLA, no LAD, OP clear, no icterus

Pul: CTAB ś W/R/R

Cor: RRR ś M/G/R

Abd: Soft, NTND, NABS ś HSM

Ext: No C/C/E

Okay, what I actually said was: "Apply one drop to both eyes once or twice daily and at bedtime as needed."

The physical examination is translated to the following:

In general, there was no apparent distress noted. Head, eyes ears, nose, and throat examination revealed normocephalic, atraumatic head. Pupils were equally reactive round and reactive to light and accommodation. There was no lymphadenopathy. Oropharynx was clear without icterus. The lung examination revealed that auscultation was clear with good airflow without wheezing, rales, or rhonchi. The heart exam showed a heart with regular rate and rhythm, no murmurs, gallops, or rubs were appreciated. The abdominal exam was soft on palpation. No tenderness or distention was appreciated. The bowel sounds were normal. No hepatomegaly was appreciated. Extremity exam showed no cyanosis, clubbing, or edema of either extremity.

Here's one thing that would happen if I didn't use abbreviations: I would spend a large proportion of my time writing and less time doing more important things like seeing patients. I already spend a very large proportion of my day writing. Even with an electronic medical records system, I still write quite a bunch. Consequently, my handwriting legibility decreases exponentially by the amount my carpal tunnel syndrome flares up.

Medical terminology is also used to describe very specific locations or conditions. For example, the word "icterus" describes a very specific yellowing of the sclera (the whites of the eyes) caused by an elevation of bilirubin. An abnormally high bilirubin can indicate impairment of the liver from such things as hepatitis, cirrhosis, or choledocholithiasis (gallstone stuck in the common bile duct) as some examples. Rales and rhonchi in a lung exam are very specific sounds. They are difficult to explain unless one has heard them before. Therefore a rale is a rale is a rale and a rhonchi is a rhonchi. They mean exactly what they are, and there are no good substitutes for those words. Even in my explanation of physical exam findings I use terms that are specific for very precise medical conditions, such as cirrhosis, hepatitis, and choledocholithiasis. There is no way to get around them.

The trend that I have seen since graduating medical school is this: ever so slowly medical terminology is being degraded. Every profession has its own terminology and abbreviations. Unfortunately society seems to want to pick mine apart. On many of the forms that I must complete for treatment or equipment authorizations, they specifically state that I must use common language to describe the physical findings or the diagnosis. That's akin to telling a mathematician to explain physics without using equations. The physical exam that I outlined above is a very standard normal exam and is typically the basis for my standard inpatient examination. In order to not overlook something in the history or miss a physical exam finding—I do the same things to everyone, the same way, in the same order—I also document the same way every time. I put a lot of information on that piece of paper, or electronic note, whichever the case may be. It is there so that I can refer back to it and know exactly what I did and saw. Three years from now when I am reviewing that note I can look at it and know exactly what happened.

Medical billing is a disaster, which I will discuss more in detail later. However, in basic form billing categorizes my evaluation and management of a patient (the practice of medicine) into levels of care based on what I "do." Specifically, how many problems I addressed, how detailed my examination was, how complicated my treatment plan is, and how long it took me to do all this. The way the insurance companies determine if I am telling the truth after I've sent off my billing information, because apparently I'm untrustworthy and they don't take my word for it, is through an audit of my medical records. Here's where the problem starts. If I am lucky someone who has taken a medical terminology class at the local community college will audit me. Many times I am not that lucky.

Often my note is compared to a list of "preapproved" words, and either the word is on the list or it isn't. If the word is there, I get "credit" for that, if not, then I don't. If I don't get enough "credit," then I will get paid from the insurance company at whatever level they have calculated based upon the number of "points" I get. If I have "over-coded" or billed at a rate higher than is documented on the audit, I must reimburse them for the difference. This is regardless of the actual amount of work that I did, just what is documented. If I "under-code," then that's just too bad for me. Physicians routinely under-code the bill.[63] I have my reasons for under-coding. The first is that an audit requires a significant amount of my staff manpower in terms of financial cost per hour as well the loss of a productive individual while they pull charts and gather the required information. Additionally if I trigger an audit from the insurance company because my billing codes are at a higher rate than my peers, and I am incorrectly over-coding, then I have to pay back the difference. That's hard to do when I've already spent that money months ago on my staff's salary. Or worse, I go to jail for insurance fraud.[64]

Regarding abbreviations, let's take my respiratory examination as an example.

"Pul: CTAB ṡ W/R/R" is fourteen characters with a very specific meaning. Specifically it means, "The lung examination revealed that auscultation was clear with good airflow without wheezing, rales, or rhonchi." This is ninety-six characters long with the same meaning. My carpal tunnel and my schedule certainly appreciate the shorter version. Unfortunately the abbreviated exam will earn me zero "points." Even if I am audited by a nurse case manager (which happened not too long ago) who knows the terminology; I still do not get credit for it.

My hospital also has a list, based upon the guidelines required by its credentialing agency, of unapproved abbreviations. These include the abbreviation "qd" for "daily" as one example. The rationale for this is, understandably, to decrease medication and order errors.[65,66] However, I do find it ironic that the government agencies that dictate that I cannot use abbreviation is notoriously riddled with its own obscure and ridiculous acronyms. For example, the CMS website alone has well over 4,400 acronyms or abbreviations.[67] Do as I say, not as I do.

On my hospital ward, the least educated person there is the ward clerk. Please do not confuse education with intelligence. I'm saying educated. It is the ward clerk's responsibility to transcribe the physician's order for type of medication, dosage, and times to be given into the hospital's computer system. Right away there's a problem. Clonidine and Klonopin (clonazepam) look very similar if one wasn't very aware that they are very different medications. That one wasn't taught in medical terminology class. Although the advent of now mandatory computerized physician order entry in the hospital setting is meant to alleviate this problem, in my corner of the world it's at a cost of millions of dollars for the hospital.[68] Seems to me the more practical and cost effective solution would to ensure at least minimum competence for those transcribing the orders. Rather than making me spell out every word in plain language in manner that a high school graduate (who is my ward clerk) can understand, how about train them? I have to be licensed and credentialed to write the orders; they should be certified to be able to take the orders off. Don't dummy down the practice of medicine. Fix the deficiencies through education. My ward clerk is quite intelligent. If she were trained then she would have no difficulties. Unfortunately medicine in general is on the edge of the slippery slope described by Kurt Vonnegut in his story "Harrison Bergeron".[69]

"Harrison Bergeron" is a futuristic story in which the agents of the Handicapper General (H-G men, or is that HVAP/JCAHO —the CMS approved credentialing agencies?) go about making everyone the same, enforcing the constitutional amendments of equality. Unfortunately, equal means below average in intelligence, strength, and ability. People are made equal by devices, which include weights to stunt speed and strength, masks to hide beauty, and thick glasses to obscure sight. Radio transmitters implanted in the ears of intelligent people emit sharp noises to prevent sustained thought. Is this the future of medicine? Will I be regulated such that I can no longer have free thought and action? You may think that this is overreaching and preposterous, but it is closer to reality than you may think.

I think I need a beer. At the very least get back on task, that is, talking about beer—I mean medicine.

# Medicine 101

Okay, so now we have heard from me numerous times that the basic premise of medicine is simply the evaluation and management of a patient by a physician. Note that I didn't say provider. Again, we can dilute down medicine at a later date. Right now we are trying to understand what those words even mean. Afterward we can talk about how much it costs and how to screw it up.

What is medicine? I am a residency trained, board certified family practitioner fully licensed in my state to practice unlimited medicine. That implies that floating around in my noggin is sufficient knowledge of basic life science, pathophysiology, anatomy, chemistry, pharmacology, and clinical experience to evaluate and manage a disease state or health status. What does that mean?

Let's start with the doctor-patient relationship. The doctor-patient relationship should be an agreement between a patient and a doctor. The doctor should, to the best of his ability, do the following:

- Make decisions that are in the best interest of the patient's health and wellbeing. These decisions may not be the answer that the patient wants to hear, however. A good example that I see almost daily is that of the individual who seeks narcotic pain medication or anti-anxiety medications for other than prescribed uses. There is certainly a time and a place for these medications, but if the patient is going to go home and misuse, abuse, or sell the medication, then obviously that is not in his or her best interest from a medical perspective. To make a decision in the patient's best interest means to weigh all the possible options and determine which option or options are acceptable solutions to the problem at hand. This may take the form of determining which medication is better or which treatment is more preferred. This sometimes becomes clouded when the physician has a personal stake in the treatment. For example, if a physician stands to gain financially from obtaining a particular diagnostic study or treatment plan, then it can become quite problematic. After all, doctors are human and still subject to stressors and temptations just like everyone else. Stark Law has significantly curbed the opportunities of physicians for financial gain from ancillary treatments or diagnostic studies, but this has come at a very high price for the health care industry as a whole, which I will discuss a bit later as I talk about survival.

- Weigh the risks and benefits of treatment or the withholding of treatment and have a discussion with the patient. Physicians are human. Sometimes it is difficult to realize that more treatment is not always the best treatment. We must look at the patient as a whole, taking into account quality of life, patient preference, cultural differences, and financial cost. The prolongation of life at the expense of quality is not always in the best interest of the patient, nor is expensive treatments that do not have a clear advantage over more conservative methods.

- Educate the patient on disease processes or the healthy lifestyle. The patient is ultimately responsible for his or her own health. Let me repeat this again as this is another very important and testable item. The patient is ultimately responsible for his or her own health. I cannot make you eat better, exercise, and quit smoking. I cannot go to your house and make sure you take your medicine promptly at 10:00 p.m. Poor lifestyle choices or choices made with incomplete or biased information is not in the best interest of the patient. In my residency there was a physician who, based upon her own personal beliefs, would not discuss birth control methods. She would not discuss it, prescribe it, or refer anyone to a physician who would. I certainly understand that there are cultural and religious differences in America. I too have my own personal beliefs, and sometimes these beliefs are in conflict with the beliefs of the patient. However, it is my charge to work for the best interest of the patient, even if that conflicts with my personal choices. Summarily, I also have the right as an American citizen to not do something that I do not believe in. If I do not perform a particular procedure or prescribe a particular medication, then I will still educate the patient; often I will explain why I am in conflict. It is ultimately the choice of the patient to seek medical care elsewhere if he or she wishes to pursue further treatment, but at least I have done my duty to educate.

- Be an advocate for the patient. Being a patient advocate does not, however, mean that I am the surrogate parent of the patient. I cannot make someone do something they are unwilling to do nor take a medication they do not wish to take or cannot afford. It is my responsibility to educate them, give them treatment options if available, and discuss the risks and benefits of various treatments versus risks if no treatment is pursued. It is ultimately the responsibility of the patient to make the final decision. I can educate them and steer them in what I feel is the most appropriate direction, but they must agree to it at the end of the day. Being an advocate means working for the best interest of the patient. This is represented in my practice usually my staff or me fighting insurance companies for authorization for diagnostic studies, treatments, or payments for services. Sometimes, however, it can mean standing up to the patient's family if it is in the patient's best interest to do so. Some family members of some patients are unfortunately not looking out for the best interest of my patient, as demonstrated by elder abuse or neglect, for example.

- Be compassionate. Very few individuals ever see me because they want to. Most are sick, have chronic diseases that we are managing together, or are there for a preventative examination so that they may try to avoid seeing me for disease management in the future. I certainly understand that, and as such do enjoy occasionally having some small fun with this.

Me: "Good Morning, Mr. Jones. Good to see you again. How are you doing?"

Mr. Jones: "Good morning. I'm doing just fine, thanks. Actually, no, if I was doing fine I wouldn't be here to see you."

Me: "Oh, I know, that was a trick question. Whatcha got going on today?"

# Insurance Companies

Let me discuss my experience with insurance companies by starting out by saying that I don't understand a thing about insurance companies. I trained in a military residency, and my first four years of practice was on active duty. I received no education regarding the insurance process, either formal or informal. In my training, I saw the patient, I treated them to the best of my ability, and I wrote a note in the patient's medical record so that I could understand in the future what I did and what I was thinking at that particular moment. I really have no idea how they (insurance companies) work on a corporate level, so let me explain the system, as I understand it on a personal level.

The purpose of medical insurance, it seems to me, is pay for the medical bills of the customers who buy the insurance. That's how my car insurance works, so I would expect that medical insurance would work similarly. I have a great car insurance company, by the way. I pay a monthly premium to the company. The insurance company, in turn, takes my money plus the premiums of a bunch of other people, invest it, and when or if something happens, they use the money they invested to pay the expenses that I have incurred. Granted, if I prove to my insurance company that I tend to be more expensive than my peers, either through being a higher risk individual or having multiple payouts, they understandably raise my rates accordingly. I understand that, and I do not begrudge them for doing so. After all, the company as a whole must remain solvent. At the end of the year, if my car insurance has made a profit for the year after expenses, it will send me a rebate check for my proportion of the difference. For example, I just received a check for about sixty dollars this year from my company for the amount of profit made from appropriately investing my premium. Sweet.

Medical insurance should provide the ability to pay for my medical costs should I need them. These costs include such things as physician office visits, medications, hospital costs, surgeries, medical equipment, and long-term care. My experience as both an American with health insurance and as a physician who is entrenched in the system is this: Health Care in America is at least three times more expensive than it needs to be, insurance companies receive significantly more revenue than they pay out to customers, and the entire system as a whole is fraught with abuse and fraud. Let me explain.

By law, in my state I must charge no more or less than what is considered "usual and customary."[70] Now, that's pretty vague, and I'm not quite sure what that even works out to be in dollar amounts. Generally speaking though, I do know that it means that I have to charge everyone the same regardless of payment type. If you have insurance I have to charge you the same as I would if you didn't have health insurance. I know what I "charge" and what I "receive," but I don't know how that equals the term "usual and customary." My experience in this regard is limited to what I remember as a child and what I experience when I go get a haircut, oil changed, or plumbing fixed.

As a kid it was rare that I went to the doctor. I had to be pretty sick or broken to go. I don't know if this was because my family didn't have insurance growing up or because the culture was different then. However, when I did go, the doctor would see me, write a prescription or an order, and we would get medicine or medical equipment (such as crutches) either at the local pharmacy or there in his office. My mother paid the bill at the time of service and in cash (or in trade sometimes if we couldn't afford the bill. I'm pretty sure I got a school sports physical for the price of a picnic lunch once), and off I went. If I needed labs or X-rays, we would take the order to the hospital, get the study, and would then get a bill a week or two later. We would pay it with cash, because it wasn't outrageously expensive, and move on with our life. Unfortunately the law/system does not allow me to do that today. A haircut will demonstrate that point.

When I get a haircut a couple of things happen. She cuts my hair over light flirting, and then I pay her for my haircut. I don't think hair stylists have the same code of ethics that I have, by the way. Anyway, what she charges me is the combination of her overhead expense plus the income she expects to make. That doesn't sound too difficult. The same holds true with my mechanic and plumber, except the flirting part, that is. They provide a service, which is calculated as business overhead plus personal income, and I pay it at the time of service.

Medicine does not do that. I have overhead. I have a lot of overhead, as a matter of fact. My overhead is in the tune of about forty-five to fifty dollars per patient in today's economy. That sounds like a bunch, and it really is. Unfortunately, there is no way that I can decrease it. I am in a seven-provider practice. We have about forty-five support staff. That's a very large amount of people. The days of a single doctor with one nurse and one receptionist are over. I need a couple of front office people to check in the patient, verify insurance company benefits, collect co-pays, and make appointments. I need one person whose sole job is insurance company interface such as authorization for treatment, medicine prior authorizations, and filling out forms. I have two assistants to actually interact with the patient when he or she is in the office. With mandatory computerized medical records and reporting requirements, my speed at which I can bring a patient from the waiting room to the exam room has slowed to a crawl, requiring me to have multiple assistants to do this. I have an entire billing and collecting team who are degreed in billing and collecting. It has become that complicated. We share an office manager, employ a full-time computer guy (information technology or IT), and we have a diagnostic department because we are remote from the hospital. That all adds up. Oh yeah, and I actually would like to pay my personal bills. I do enjoy eating and have to put gas in my car. I also had to buy all the equipment that I used, including the X-ray, CT, and ultrasound machines. That puts my personal debt burden at about 1.2 million dollars. The electronic medical records system that CMS says is mandatory alone was about a quarter million dollars for the office.

So that brings me back to the cost of health care at the most basic level, which is at the interface of the primary care doctor and patient. When my practice was still privately owned, we used to have to negotiate our own rates with the insurance companies. In a nutshell, we expected to get from the insurance company approximately one third of what our charges were. So, for example, if we charged one hundred dollars for something, we could expect about thirty-three dollars or so back, depending on what we were doing. I'm going to use the one hundred dollar example a fair amount throughout. The reason is because it's a good approximation of my average charges per encounter, and for this biology major it's easy to do the math.

So right away there's a problem. If the insurance company on average pays me about one third of my charges, and my average charge is about one hundred dollars, I can expect about thirty-three bucks back. Wait a minute, but my overhead alone is forty-five dollars. That means that if I extend this example to my hair stylist, she is paying out fifteen dollars every time I get my hair cut. I'm pretty sure she would not stay in business very long at that rate no matter how cute she is.

But we aren't talking about her. We are talking about me. That's what I am making. And yet I am expected to continue to do this, no, wait. I am supposed to work for less than that. For some reason in America there is a perception that paying medical bills is optional. There is a threefold reason for this based on my experience. The first reason is that back in the days when medicine was profitable, i.e. not now, primary care physicians worked with an actual profit margin. That meant that they didn't have to collect 100 percent of what they charged to stay afloat financially. Doctors, at least primary care, as a general rule do what we do not because we expect to get rich doing it.

I had a medical assistant once who was married to a union plumber. On any given day, her husband made more money per hour than I ever did. He didn't make more annually, but only because I worked three times more actual hours than he did. However, on an hour per hour basis, he made more than I did. I'm also not talking about being "on call." Doctors like to say that we are "always working" because we are "always on call" or some such nonsense. There are plenty of other jobs out there with similar or more hourly requirements than mine. My dad worked twelve-hour shifts seven days a week. Once every two weeks he would get a day off. I promise you I don't work that much. I will clock in sixty or so hours in the office and another twenty to thirty answering my phone all night, but it's not what my dad did. I can't complain about that.

Anyway, back when medicine was profitable, doctors had the luxury of not having to scrap for every penny they charged. We are humanitarians by nature. We like to help people. Even the sub-subspecialists with the really big egos at the end of the day like to help people. That's why we do what we do. Back then we could write off a bill or two. If you didn't pay your bill, then it didn't matter quite so much. Plus since we usually were our own business managers, we didn't really know any better. A lot of things fell through the cracks. They don't teach us accounting in medical school. Doctors tend to be poor businessmen. Hearts are too big maybe.

Fast forward to today. My overhead is forty-five dollars. I charge one hundred dollars and expect to get back about thirty-three dollars. Don't think I'm not going to hunt you down if you don't pay your bill.

Secondly, there's a perception that doctors are "rich," and if you are paying your bill, all you are really doing is paying for my Fiji vacation or my yacht payment. Regarding primary care, I will refer back to the plumber analogy. Granted, I am not talking about surgical subspecialists such as cardiothoracic surgeons or neurosurgeons. But then again, they can have that job, no thanks.

Finally there's the perception that the insurance company will take care of it all and the patient (you) don't have to pay anything else. This is a bit more troublesome, and this is where the system falls apart.

I will stand before you and make the statement that in America the average person seeking medical care pays at least three times for the same service. As a matter of fact, I make this statement almost every single day when I explain insurance companies to my patients.

First, let's start with the insurance premium. I don't know how they calculate it, but I do know it's friggin expensive, almost $16,000 for a family.[71] I really don't know what they do with all that money. If it were not spent on executive bonuses and investor dividends, would it continue to be so expensive? So, on average a patient spends about ten grand a year plus or minus based on my experience. Barring catastrophe, that's money that is for all practical purposes thrown away. You will never see that money again. Bye bye, Uncle Benjamin. That's squeeze number one.

Now, let's take the average American in my office. Obese, diabetic, hypertensive, high cholesterol. Even with all that, four to six doctor visits a year plus labs and an occasional diagnostic study equals somewhere between $2,500 to $3,500 a year.

Hmm, according to my front office people the average deductible paid is somewhere between $2,500 to $3,500. That means that even though you are paying twelve large every year, you still have to basically pay cash above and beyond your insurance premium for everything I do to you in a calendar year. That's squeeze number two.

If I charge one hundred dollars, and the contracted allowable that I have negotiated with your insurance company is only thirty-three dollars, then at the end of the day I have to make up the fifteen-dollar difference somewhere, assuming I want to eat this week. It will be twenty bucks if I want to put gas in my car. Thanks to Pete Stark and the Stark laws, my ability to make this up in ancillary services, also called designated health services, is very limited. As per CMS.gov:

Section 1877 of the Social Security Act (the Act) (42 U.S.C. 1395nn), also known as the physician self-referral law and commonly referred to as the "Stark Law"[72] states:

- Prohibits a physician from making referrals for certain designated health services (DHS) payable by Medicare to an entity with which he or she (or an immediate family member) has a financial relationship (ownership, investment, or compensation), unless an exception applies.

- Prohibits the entity from presenting or causing to be presented claims to Medicare (or billing another individual, entity, or third party payer) for those referred services.

- Establishes a number of specific exceptions and grants the Secretary the authority to create regulatory exceptions for financial relationships that do not pose a risk of program or patient abuse.

The following items or services are DHS:

- Clinical laboratory services.
- Physical therapy services.

- Occupational therapy services.

- Outpatient speech-language pathology services.

- Radiology and certain other imaging services.

- Radiation therapy services and supplies.

- Durable medical equipment and supplies.

- Parenteral and enteral nutrients, equipment, and supplies.

- Prosthetics, orthotics, and prosthetic devices and supplies.

- Home health services.

- Outpatient prescription drugs.

- Inpatient and outpatient hospital services.

Okay, so how do I make up the difference? I can't reduce my overhead, because CMS had mandated that I must meet "Meaningful Use" for electronic medical records or it will start reducing my payments. My IT guy, for example, makes a decent salary without contributing in a positive way to the revenue stream. I can't invest in ancillary services, because Pete Stark says I can't. I have only two options: increase my fee schedule and/or see more patients.

My fee schedule is limited to "usual and customary." In today's market, "usual and customary" is a little more than three times more than what it should actually cost. Why? Because I average only about a third of what I charge through contractual agreements. I'm shooting for that magical forty-five dollars. I can't make up the difference in ancillary services thanks to Stark law, so my only source of income is office visits. That automatically drives my cost up to a hundred and twenty dollars or so. After all, a barber won't cut your hair for less than it costs her, but I should? Either way, that's my overhead cost (still not talking about my personal income, just my business expense). Here comes squeeze number three. I have to charge everyone the same regardless of payment status. If you do not have insurance, then I am charging you the same as if you had insurance, especially Medicare. That's about one hundred to a hundred and twenty dollars. Ouch. That's pretty steep for something that really should only be costing you about thirty-five dollars. Of course given the IT guy and the extra staff I have to have, it ends up being about fifty-five dollars, but that's still cheaper than a hundred and twenty dollars. On average, for an average office visit you have paid approximately three hundred big ones while your insurance company have paid out little to nothing.

So in a nutshell, you pay three times for your health care. And that's just in my office. It gets a lot worse in the hospital and specialist offices. But really, is a heart bypass worth a half million? I guess that depends on whether or not it's your heart. I guess also whether or not you are part of the "health care industry." Does an HR manager or VP of something-or-other contribute to the actual care of any individual patient? Guess that depends on whether or not you are the manager or VP and feel threatened. Remember the basics. Medicine is the evaluation and management of a patient by a physician. A nurse carries out the care orders of the physician. The therapists carry out the therapy order of the physician. The pharmacist prepares the medications ordered by the physician. All ancillary services are secondary to the evaluation and management of the patient by the physician. Unfortunately, they all take a cut. Throw in human resources, legal, custodial services, maintenance, and administrative support, and imagine where all the health care dollars are going—definitely not to me. I won't be vacationing in Fiji anytime soon. Makes a picnic lunch seem cheap. Did I say I think health care for trade is illegal? I don't think a chicken dinner is considered a usual and customary fee.

Speaking of squeezing the system, how much income generated, in dollars, by health insurance companies goes toward "administrative costs?" In 2010 the federal government passed the Patient Protection and Coverage Act, which requires 80 to

85 percent of premiums goes toward payment of medical claims. That's a start, but when the numbers are in the billions of dollars, that's still a chunk of change that isn't getting spent on your health care. Gross revenue for Humana Inc. in 2011 according to their 2011 Annual Report was $36,832,000,000 ($36.8 billion). Go to Louisville and look at the Humana Building. What is the overhead cost of that puppy? How many people work there? How much does the CEO make? Is it more than any single physician in its network? Of course it is. Look at these numbers:

### Insurance Company CEO Total Compensation 2011:[73]

- Cigna, David Cordani: $19,100,000

- UnitedHealth, Stephen Hemsley: $13,400,000

- Wellpont, Angela Braly: $13,300,000

- Health Care Service Group, Patricia Hemingway Hall: $12,900,000

- Aetna, Mark Bertolini: 10,600,000

- Humana, Michael McCallister: $7,300,000

How much is administrative support worth? It appears obviously a bunch. How much is the ability to save your life worth? Apparently it's not nearly that much. Median total income for primary care was $212,840 and for specialists $384,467. For the full report on physician compensation, be prepared to pay $625 for the MGMA publication *Physician Compensation and Production Survey 2012 Report Based on 2011 Data.*

With the Patient Protection and Coverage Act, 80 to 85 percent of premiums are supposed to go toward payment of medical claims, leaving 15 to 20 percent attributed to "administrative expenses." To me, that is still an astronomically large amount of money. Even if you give the CEO of Humana his 0.5 percent of the net revenue, that's still something like 7.3 billion dollars that doesn't have to be spent on claims. Again, do they really have 7 billion dollars in overhead annually? When I am scrapping to negotiate fifty cents or a dollar more per office visit, and the net income reported in the 2011 annual report is $1.4 billion (presumably after "administrative expenses") these kinds of operating margins leave a bitter taste.

Morally, I have issue with this. I would think a conscientious insurance company should strive to operate at net revenue of zero. If they are making money, then that money needs to either be invested into the future of the company to ensure solvency or returned to the customers. There should be no reason why an insurance company should have a net income in the billions. Even if a CEO needs to be a multi-millionaire (which I find debatable) does that justify financially raping the populous? If you are having chest pain, is a CEO more important than a cardiologist? Or more importantly, more vital than a family physician for that matter, the front line of medicine? I'm the guy who must understand on the most basic and comprehensive level everything that is going on with you and decide if you need to see the cardiologist in the first place. Ironically, the only other specialty that is compensated even less than I are the pediatricians who specialize in taking care of our future, our children. Unfortunately, these days I'm preoccupied with whether your insurance plan will pay me that extra fifty cents or dollar for the evaluation of your chest pain.

I can only hope that the health insurance premiums that I pay as a consumer are being invested wisely to ensure the future solvency of the insurance company. I have noticed that, since the advent of the partial adoption of health care reform, insurance premiums and deductibles have increased significantly, while insurance companies are paying out less at the primary care office level. This sounds suspiciously familiar:

> A Ponzi scheme is an investment fraud that involves the payment of purported returns to existing investors from funds contributed by new investors. Ponzi scheme organizers often solicit new investors by promising to invest

funds in opportunities claimed to generate high returns with little or no risk. [AKA health care coverage]. In many Ponzi schemes, the fraudsters focus on attracting new money to make promised payments to earlier-stage investors and to use for personal expenses, instead of engaging in any legitimate investment. With little or no legitimate earnings, the schemes require a consistent flow of money from new investors to continue. Ponzi schemes tend to collapse when it becomes difficult to recruit new investors or when a large number of investors ask to cash out [AKA get old].

Abuse and fraud is everywhere. I tell my children that America is founded on two basic principles. The first is that we do not play well with others. Europeans originally migrated to America because we did not get along with the establishment. Pick your example. The pilgrims were a religious sect, and the founding fathers have been described as anarchists.[74,75] The second is that America is based on the premise of exploitation of others. That lesson I learned in college sociology as I learned about the influential American families of the 19th century and watching the Rachel Maddow Show via her coverage of politics.

That pervasive attitude is still alive and well. If there is a buck to be made on the exploitation of the "system," then we as Americans will find it. It is estimated that somewhere near 10 percent, which amounts annually to around 150 billion dollars, of all health care expenditures are due to fraud or abuse.[76] Some glaring examples that I see are home health care and durable medical equipment.

Home health is necessary when a patient is discharged from the hospital but needs specialized care. This may include skilled nursing care or home therapy. This home health care must be justified and ordered by a physician. I have personally seen examples where the discharging hospital has automatically initiated home health care services without the order of the physician.

Sometime later I receive a faxed document requiring my signature for the services rendered. If it's buried amongst the forty other things I have to sign first thing in the morning before I start my day, it gets lost and is usually signed without too much questioning. After all, we are supposed to be a "team" working for the best interest of the patient. The net result is the patient may have received services that were unnecessary. Or, as I saw recently, services were trying to be rendered on a patient who had been dead for many months. The same holds true for durable medical equipment such as home oxygen supplies and mobility devices like walkers, wheelchairs, and motorized scooters.

In the attempt to curb fraud and abuse, CMS has imposed a rule that all ancillary services including durable medical equipment require a face-to-face examination between the patient and me as well as written justification as to the need for the equipment or service. Although this increases my already overloaded workload and I groan at the additional work, I do appreciate the intention of the law. By forcing the responsibility of deciding what services and equipment are needed on the physician in a face-to-face encounter, it enforces and supports the physician-patient relationship.

That brings me back to the hundred-dollar office visit. We assumed that the insurance company was even going to pay us in the first place. They are masters at finding excuses to not pay for services rendered or dictate care based upon coverage. Here are some common reasons in my office:

Step therapy. Step therapy is an algorithmic approach in which a provider would start or try one medication as first line. If the patient does not show clinical improvement on this medication, the medication is changed or another medication is added. In a "textbook perfect" patient this works well. The classic example is that of asthma. According to an "expert panel," the "proper treatment" of asthma has been clearly defined. If patients meet the requirements for a diagnosis of mild intermittent asthma, it is recommended that they use a short-acting inhaler that reduces airway spasm (bronchodilator), such as albuterol. If the asthma is worse and they meet the diagnosis of persistent asthma, then additional medications, such as inhaled steroids and long-acting bronchodilators, are used. Other medications are added in sequence as the severity of the disease worsens. That sounds fine in theory if everyone follows the textbook. However, since practicing medicine is akin to being a mechanic where every car is a different make and model and there is no owner's manual, as a family physician I must get creative when treating patients.

That's the art of medicine. Many patients also have other medical or social problems, which complicate treatment. Also, not every medication is used precisely as FDA approved. The skills that I have learned in my training have allowed me to understand pathophysiology as well as pharmacology, and my experience as a physician has taught me to navigate through the socioeconomic quagmire. Therefore, I may use a medication in a novel way that may not be FDA approved. It is my job and responsibility to understand what I am doing and to treat the patient to the best of my ability. Many medications are used in this manner. It is called "off-label" use. By fully understanding the basic science of medicine we are able to use the tools available to us as physicians to find the best treatment for the patient.

Unfortunately, this often conflicts with the rigid algorithmic approach. An example is a patient I saw today. This was an eighty-year-old female who had Influenza A four weeks ago. She presented to me with a continued dry cough and shortness of breath after fits of coughing. After appropriate evaluation and a normal chest X-ray to rule out pneumonia, I decided that she has an acute inflammatory process of her large airways, secondary to her recent influenza, which I affectionately call reactive bronchitis. By further understanding the basic pathophysiology and taking into consideration her age and other medical problems, called co-morbidities, I decided that she would most benefit from

a combination inhaled steroid to relieve the inflammation as well as a long-acting bronchodilator to also relieve any possible constriction of her airway from muscle contraction. She did not feel better after a trial of a short-acting bronchodilator in my office. As a matter of fact, it made her cough even more.

Unfortunately, due to her insurance and the rigid step therapy algorithm, she must also use a short-acting bronchodilator, even though they make her worse and she does not carry a diagnosis of asthma. Since the particular medication that I wish to use is only FDA indicated for asthma, the insurance company guidelines only refer to the algorithm. Although algorithms are good tools for aiding in the diagnosis and treatment of medical conditions, they should not be so rigidly followed as to preclude other treatment options or methods. Strict algorithms negate the individual, the doctor, evaluating the patient and considering other treatment options or diagnoses. For the straightforward and clear-cut scenarios it works, but in cases where the diagnosis is more complex or the other comorbidities must be taken into account, blindly following an algorithm becomes dangerous.

In her particular case it is the inflammation causing the symptoms rather than spasm of the airways. The medication that I prefer is prohibitively expensive for the patient; therefore unless her insurance will cover it, she cannot afford it on her fixed income. Here is what happens: I prescribe it. She takes the prescription to the pharmacy, and it is there that she finds out that her insurance will not cover it. The pharmacy sends me a fax called a prior authorization. This is a form that my assistant must fill out, which requires me to provide justification for the need for this medication. If, in the case of step therapy, she has not tried any short-acting bronchodilator or carries a diagnosis of asthma or emphysema, the medication will not be authorized. The de facto denial of coverage for a treatment modality is the practicing of medicine. After all, who now is making the decision which medication this patient will receive? The prohibitive cost of the medication is a significant barrier to health care delivery. The denial of such medication coverage is equivalent to making a decision regarding evaluation and management of the patient.

Unfortunately, the only people who seem to understand that is me and the patient it affects. If a poor outcome results from the denial of a medication by an insurance carrier, the ultimate responsibility still falls on me, even though I no longer have the ability to control which medication the patient will receive.

What is a prior authorization or precertification? Prior authorization is a misnomer implying that something can be done ahead of time. It refers to the denial of a medication or service by an insurance carrier. Medication denials are most common in my daily life. As a matter of fact, I dedicate an entire employee (at the associated increase in overall health care cost) to fighting these all day long. Some medications are just flat not covered by an insurance carrier, such as the stomach medicine I described earlier. Some are only covered if one tries "step therapy." Some insurance carriers only cover one medication in each class of medication or only if a patient fails multiple medications of the same or similar class. In this particular instance, it is very common to have the insurance carrier refuse to tell me what medication in that class they will cover. They tell me that they are not authorized to release that information. I am supposed to guess which one of the six medications in that particular class they will cover. In other instances I need a "precert." A precertification is simply an approval by the insurance for a procedure or diagnostic test. Also physicians must go through clinical steps, which may not be medically necessary, in order to get the procedure or diagnostic test approved.

Precerts are not covered for any number of reasons. Mostly it is due to not documenting in the patient's chart the "keywords" necessary for approval. An example would be an MRI without a documented neurologic problem such as numbness or weakness. Another example is a test of the gallbladder called a HIDA (hepatobiliary iminodiacetic) scan, which specifically looks at how well the gallbladder is functioning. Often this is not approved without an ultrasound of the gallbladder, regardless of the results of any other diagnostic testing.

The other day, I had a thirty-two-year-old male patient come into my office with a complaint of back pain. I obtained my history and performed my examination. He had, based on my history and physical examination, a classic or "textbook" case of nerve impingement in his back. If I were to open my medical school textbook and read about nerve impingement, I would have not been surprised if I saw his picture there. Unfortunately, since this was the first time I had seen this particular patient, I had no previous tests or exams. There are many ways to treat this particular problem. Some treatment options include physical therapy, anti-inflammatory medication or muscle relaxers, steroid injections, or in severe cases surgery. The treatment plan is determined by the anatomy of the patient, in other words what is wrong anatomically, and the response of the patient to previous treatment.

In this case, the patient would have benefitted from first-line physical therapy. It is not a covered service on his insurance. He can't afford to pay out-of-pocket for it, and he can't take off work three days a week anyway. In my limited time I teach him basic stretching, give him a booklet reinforcing these maneuvers, prescribe an anti-inflammatory and a muscle relaxer for any spasm he may be having, and cross my fingers.

He returns the next week in significantly worse pain. Now he is having not only leg pain but also weakness. I am pretty confident at this time, based upon my examination, that he has a disk that is pushing on a nerve. He has failed as much conservative treatment as I can do. Now I need to know anatomy. The most straightforward test that I have in my repertoire is an MRI. I could do an X-ray, but it would not show soft tissue, such as a bulging disk. I could do a CT scan, but the image quality on a CT would not be nearly as good as an MRI, and although I could get a decent idea of what is going on, if it was abnormal then I would have to get a more definitive test. I could do a nerve conduction study called an electromyelogram or EMG, which would determine if he were having disruption of the nerve conduction. Based on his numbness and weakness that I could see clinically, I already knew the answer to that question. I needed to see his soft tissue anatomy so I could determine what direction I needed to go.

I attempt to get an MRI. The first question asked of my assistant trying to get approval was, "What other studies has he had?" The answer was of course none. Up until now diagnostic imaging was not indicated. I am done. Without some sort of other diagnostic imaging, I cannot hope to get an MRI. I get a plain X-ray. It of course shows mild degenerative changes only. X-rays do not show nerves or disks. He is now out about a hundred and fifty dollars since this X-ray cost went to his deductible. I try to get an MRI now. The insurance company says nope, unless I want speak to the insurance company's physician for a "peer to peer" discussion, except its Friday afternoon, and he won't be back until Monday next week. What else can I do? Now that I can get something else besides an X-ray, I can get a CT scan. It isn't as good as an MRI, but if is normal then that would be useful. I get a CT scan for about a thousand dollars. It is abnormal, showing that he has evidence for significant nerve impingement. This appears, based upon the results of the CT, that he may need to see a neurosurgeon. I try to make an appointment. My assistant makes the call but informs me that we can't make the specialist appointment until he has reviewed the results of the MRI first. Back to the insurance company. I now get the MRI that I wanted originally. Unfortunately I have spent almost twelve hundred dollars of unnecessary testing. I would like to say that this is the exception, but this was an average Friday.

There are other examples of denials of coverage or payment. Some common ones we see in my office include changing claims address without communicating or updating ID cards. For an insurance claim to go through to the company and they actually pay something, everything has to match. The name of the patient must exactly match that on the card; the addresses must be correct. The patient identification number and policy numbers must be exact. Changing the address to send the claim is one method of avoiding payment. Also is changing payer ID without communicating or updating ID cards, or changing member ID number without sending the member an updated card.

Currently, insurance companies can deny coverage for conditions that occurred prior to acquiring health insurance. With the current health care reform, the ability of insurance companies to deny coverage for preexisting condition may be more difficult. Unfortunately, health care regulation is constantly in motion, and this may not be the case.

Other methods include requesting information from member/provider but never send the form to complete the requested information. Insisting that another insurance company is the primary insurance and point the finger or denying a claim by stating that the physician is not in the network, when in fact the provider is in network. Also, companies will bundle procedures by paying one flat, reduced rate for multiple procedures or reduce the payment amount if multiple procedures are done at the same time. In a primary care office often the amount of a bundled payment does not cover the overhead for the additional supplies and time.

Insurance companies will also let claims sit in their systems without being processed until we follow up on them, or state that claim information was incomplete even though we "scrub" the claim to be sure that all the required information is present and it is sent electronically.

# Exam Room Etiquette

Okay, some things seem simple and easy. Sunday mornings, getting caught in the rain, pina coladas, long walks along the beach, you get the picture. There are other things that seem simple and easy to me as a physician, but apparently some patients struggle with this. Let me help you out by outlining the obvious things you should do or not do in the exam room.[77] Although this discussion may sound a bit crass and flippant, it really does affect your overall health. After all, how eager do you think I am to interact with you if you are rude, obnoxious, or otherwise unpleasant to deal with? I have, on more than one occasion, dismissed patients from my practice simply on the basis of that. If you curse at my staff or me, or threaten in any way, I lose my ability to stay objective. If you scream at my staff over the phone and call my assistant the dreaded B word because I feel that I need to properly evaluate you in the office rather than simply call in whatever prescription you are wanting, then do not become upset when I do not invite you back to my practice. So far, that right has not been taken away from me yet.

Okay, to start, keep your paws off me. The exam room is not an appropriate place for naughty touch. Especially if you are supermodel hot; don't make me go home and cry into my pillow. I will. It's tragic. Please see my previous discussion. Doctors are not pieces of meat, despite what you see on television. This goes both ways, and I also prefer not to be front-page news in the local paper for sexual harassment. If you are of the opposite sex and I am doing anything more than shaking your hand or examining you with your clothes on, you bet your biscuit I have a chaperone. My criterion is if I can associate what I am doing with getting on a base, then I need a standby. An exception may be if I comment favorably on a piece of jewelry, such as calling your dolphin naval ring "cute" or commenting on other accoutrements not normally seen. It's not because I am hitting on you; it's because it may be legitimately a cute little dolphin. I've seen everything, and just because it's dolphin jewelry don't make it cute.

Don't complain about something if you don't want me to poke, mash, or otherwise examine it. Specifically, don't complain about something in your junk area if you don't want me checking it out. I don't know how many times I've had a conversation that sounds something like this:

Patient: "Doctor, I have this horrible pain and/or bleeding from some orifice in my junk area."

Me: "Hmm... that could be serious. Let's take a look."

Patient: "What? You want to look at my va-jay-jay?"

Me: "Yes, ma'am."

Patient: "But I don't want you to look there. Can't you just give me something for it?"

And this conversation goes on until either the patient decides that whatever it was that was bothering him/her isn't really such a big deal, or I check out the area. Believe me, it's not a big deal. Sometimes I check so many packages I think I'm working for the postal service. It's part of the job. Get over it. I did a long time ago.

Along those same lines, don't complain about something that could be serious then refuse to get evaluated. My internal lawyer throws a fit. The complaint of crushing chest pain will get you an evaluation every stinking time. As will bleeding but especially rectal bleeding/coughing up blood, shortness of breath, weak and dizzy (my personal nemesis), I can't feel my "fill in the body part," "I want to kill myself," or anything similar. I'm not going to just tell you "it's nothing to worry about," because it could be something to worry about. It could be serious or potentially life threatening. In other words, it could kill you. I don't care what your deductible is on your insurance. Nor do I care that you can't make your CAT scan appointment because you are planning to be out of town on vacation next week. If you're dead, it doesn't matter much, now does it? It's awfully hard to sip margaritas from beyond the grave.

Don't demand. It just pisses me off.

Patient: "I demand that something be done."

Me: "Sir, did you get your MRI? [or other appropriate diagnostic study]?

Patient: "No, I refuse to take that test. I can't afford it, and I was out of town on vacation that week."

Me: *So you can afford to go on vacation, but you can't afford to get this horrible pain evaluated?* "Until I know what's causing your pain, I don't know how to treat it."

Patient: "This needs to be corrected right now!"

Me: "How do you propose I do that?"

Patient: "I don't know. You're the doctor."

Me: "Without knowing what's causing the problem, I can't fix it. I recommend an MRI to look at the area."

Patient: "Well, I'm not going to do that."

Or

Me: "What you have is part of normal aging. You will have this problem, and it will probably get worse."

Patient: "You need to fix it."

Me: "It's not something I can fix. It's normal."

Patient: "I demand that something be done. I refuse to have this problem."

Me: "How about we do some testing?" *Then after your potentially expensive and probably unnecessary testing, we can discuss how I still can't fix it.*

Listen to your mother. Specifically, wash behind your ears and wear clean underwear. Remember, odds are if you are in my exam room and something is dripping, oozing, hurting, itching, or has a rash, I'm going to look at it and probably poke you with some sort of object. That's my job; that's what I do. I understand if you're very ill or in a hurry because you just got off work, but that's the exception. In my office there's a certain percentage that just have poor hygiene. Ugh, I mean really. I have to work there. Do a man a solid and scrub that.

When I was in the navy I was stationed aboard a ship. On this particular ship I was stationed aboard we had a boiler room with an ambient temperature of about 120 degrees. Countless days were spent examining these sailors after four hours of working in that heat. Both men and women, and often these exams were full physicals with all the bells and whistles, metal objects suitable for prodding, and of course the ubiquitous powdered latex gloves. I didn't mind when these sailors came to my office smelling like a goat. They had an important job to do and often were pulled into my office unexpectedly. As a general rule they were mostly clean to begin with. I can't say the same for my civilian clientele. Dirt and debris as well as bits of old food do tend to accumulate under skin folds and in dark moist areas. So do fungi such as Candida, which is a type of yeast. Unless you are making friendship bread, I strongly recommend you tackle those trouble areas with some soap and water before you wander into my office. Sometimes I can't get the smell out of my exam room, and I have to close off that room for the rest of the day.

Don't be a smartass. This is a biggie. I promise you it's not funny, and it's potentially dangerous. I'm already thirty minutes behind, have a million things to juggle in my head, and now I have to listen to your dumb ass.

Me: "What can I do for you?"

Patient: "You tell me. You're the doctor."

Me: "Okay, what's the matter? What do you have going on today?"

Patient: "If I knew that I wouldn't be here seeing you."

Me: "Why are you here?"

Patient: "You need to fix me."

Me: *Where is my baseball bat?* "It says here you have been coughing. Can you tell me about that?"

Patient: "I just told your nurse. You have all the information."

Me: *Okay, don't make me get off this stool and come over there.* "She only told me that you had a cough, and I'm not a mind reader. You're going to have to tell me what's going on so I can help you."

Needless to say, it's not humorous, and I don't appreciate it. A very large proportion, upward of 90 percent, of the information that we use to create an assessment and treatment plan comes from the history. It's very important that this part be done right. Let me explain how this process works and then how it gets screwed up.

Classically patients come in to see the doctor to take care of one or maybe two problems at a time. As a matter of fact, we encourage you to keep it to one or two problems at a time. It gets astronomically confusing to try to mentally sort, evaluate, and manage more than a couple of issues in one sitting. Plus it can get tricky from a treatment standpoint. Above all do no harm and all that. Anyway, at the start of the office visit there is usually what we call a chief complaint. This is the reason why you are here in the first place. It can be blood pressure follow up, diabetes, physical examination, pain, sickness, you name it. With every chief complaint we subsequently ask a series of questions that we call the history of present illness or HPI. These questions expand upon that initial problem, and it is from the HPI that we can paint the picture of what it is that we think is going on.

There are classically eight questions that need to be answered.[78] Using the classic example of pain, we ask the following questions:

Where does it hurt (location)? As simple as it sounds, it can be a difficult question. Answers like "all over" and "everywhere" aren't very helpful. Understandably, there are some conditions in which that answer is most appropriate, but not with a sprained ankle. I tell patients to point to the spot where it hurts with one finger. That usually helps. It also isn't always useful to give me a play by play of every discomfort you ever had since kindergarten and where it hurt. If you rolled your ankle in the 1980s and it's better now, it probably isn't pertinent.

How long have you had the pain (duration)? Again, "forever" is not very useful. That will get an involuntary eye roll. "I don't know" doesn't work either. I'm not asking to the minute, although the more precise the better, generally speaking, but give me a ballpark idea. Has that stuffy nose been going on for just a day, a week, months, or years?

What does it feel like (quality)? Kudos to all on this one for the most part. It's just what it sounds like. Crushing pain, sharp stabbing pain, pain that gradually builds up then fades, constant dull pain, whatever. You got this one; run with it.

How bad is it (severity)? I will say this only once, so pay attention. A pain of eleven on a one to ten scale is a useless statement, and it makes me want to help you find a new doctor. If you can sit in the exam room and text your friends while whining about how long it took me to get in the room to see you, then it's not an eleven. A ten is the most severe pain you have ever had. Gunshot wound maybe; leg bone poking out through your jeans will get you a ten in my book. The virtual wounds that I want to inflict upon you with my baseball bat are still only about a seven or eight, not an eleven.

When do you have it (timing)? Not too difficult to screw up. All the time? Sure. Only with sex? Absolutely. On Tuesdays at noon? Okay. Sounds fine. Just answer the question.

What makes it better or worse (exacerbating/alleviating)? With a little coaching, that's pretty straightforward. At this point I'll usually just throw out some possibilities and try to narrow it down just like a psychic friend. I start general and work toward more specific depending on the answers I get.

In what context do you have it (associated with eating, for example)? That's very similar to the above question, and I typically roll those together.

Do you have anything else that goes with it (associated features)? This one is all over the place and can be difficult from both the doctor's and the patient's perspective. Is that right shoulder pain that you're having associated at all with that abdominal pain you have after you eat? If you have gallstones you bet your biscuit it does. Is that neck pain that you have related to the chest pain you have when you walk to the mailbox? Sure. Is that rash associated with your joint pain? Maybe, maybe not. When in doubt just throw it out there, and I can sift through it pretty quickly.

From those basic questions we can usually get a fairly good idea of what we think could be causing the problem. Unfortunately, this list can be a long one depending on what you come in with and how much information I get from you. If you don't tell me everything then I can't rule out certain conditions, and at the same time if you tell me too much, I have to add in additional possibilities. This is a tricky part of the process and requires a good relationship between you and your doctor and good communication skills on both sides. Obviously it gets easier when the appointment is for a follow up on a chronic condition or even if I have a good relationship with the patient. Together we can efficiently but thoroughly work the HPI together.

I will be the first to admit that some doctors are horrible at communication. I would like to believe that I am not necessarily one of them, but I know they are out there. I hear about it all the time. People often complain to me about other doctors they saw whose mastery of the English language was exceptionally poor, they were rude and/or obnoxious, or they didn't listen. That last one is a biggie.

Once upon a time I had a crusty old doctor tell me that if I could only do one thing right, that would be to learn to listen to what my patients are telling me. Now in retrospect I don't know if he was giving me good advice or implying that I was an idiot and there was no hope that I could ever actually learn anything technically useful. I would like to think that on that day his office was his dojo and he was passing his wisdom down to me before sending me out into the world with my mad ninja medical skills. That's how I took it anyway. As little as 7 percent of human com-munication is through spoken words. The remaining 97 percent is nonverbal such as body language, pitch and tone of voice, and eye contact.[79] If I don't get the listening part down, then I am missing the vast majority of what is being told to me. The tricky part is learning to do this quickly.

In my office I don't have the luxury of time. As a matter of fact, time is absolutely the most precious commodity. I wish I had thirty minutes to sit with every patient and bond. However, in family practice there is literally no margin anywhere. One of the net results of dwindling payments is that my appointment times are ten minutes long. That gives me about twenty seconds from the time I walk into your exam room to read you. That makes body language very important.

As part of my training as a second year medical student we were formally taught how to obtain a history and physical exami-nation. For our final examination one of the things we had to do was to interview mock patients. These were staff members and volunteers who presented with certain problems. We had to obtain an adequate history using the questions that are part of the HPI, and we had to do an examination that was appropriate for the chief complaint. I breezed through all but one of these.

The mock patient presented to me a chief complaint of fatigue. He just didn't feel well. He was sitting on the examination table with his head down. He made little to no eye contact with me, and his answers were vague and short. I went through my list of questions and did a general examination based on the very little information that I found. Having not really found anything objective, my assessment was generalized malaise and my proposed plan was some lab testing and a follow-up appointment. The preceptor in the room asked me if there was anything else that I wanted to do, and I told him that I was done with my exam. The instructor then proceeded to complete the scenario by saying that by the time the patient's follow-up appointment time had arrived the patient had committed suicide. Although I was technically correct in everything I did, I wasn't listening to the patient. I didn't see that he was depressed. I was only listening to his words and not listening to the other 93 percent of what he was telling me. That was seventeen years ago. I still think about that scenario when I go into an exam room. Always listen.

On the other hand, that doesn't give you a green light to bombard me with a bunch of stupid stuff. Remember, your health depends on me clearly understanding what you are telling me. In the 1980s there was a study done that said that on average patients were interrupted eighteen seconds into explaining their problems.[80] I remember when that came out. It seemed to me that doctors were vilified as insensitive and inconsiderate. Although there are some with whom this may apply, I am just struggling to get useful information out of what you are telling me. Remember I am trying to answer the eight primary questions of the HPI, which can be very easy or a pain in the ass depending on your level of cooperation. I know this is a fine balance, and at the end of the day there is no right answer. Too much information, too little information, the wrong kind of information–all these scenarios affect my ability to absorb and process the information that I am receiving. To say that there is an exact and proper way is hubris. Instead I just ask that we all, including me, remain aware of the pitfalls of information gathering. This is where I enjoy the list. Write it down, type it up, whichever, and then hand me the list. Don't read it to me. Just write down what it is you want me to know. I can assimilate the information very quickly, determine what we need to address, and I have a record that I can scan into my computer system for reference later if need be. If it is read, then that is usually associated with the need to explain and expound on what is written. If I have questions I will ask.

Since I'm on the topic, there are other ways in which we make communication difficult. I'll start with what I see, then with what I hope I don't do.

The two-fer: that's short for two for one, two patients in the same room. Granted, a lot of the time it's two kids with similar problems, but sometimes it isn't. It's often complicated trying to keep it straight. A variation on the two-fer, the husband/wife combo, is the pinnacle of two-fer frustration. My experience is they talk at the same time at and to each other. They don't remember who had what and often conflict each other. It is also not uncommon for the wife to do all the talking while the husband is simply not allowed to join the conversation. I have found that this can be very detrimental. Many times the husband has problems that he does not want to discuss in front of his wife, such as depression, or that dull achy chest pain that he has been having for the past few months because he doesn't want his wife to overreact or to scare her. I try to separate the spouses whenever possible for that very reason.

The "oh, by the way": if you have more than one problem that you want to discuss, please tell me up front. I have ten minutes.

Don't waste it all on a hangnail and then as I am walking out of the exam room go, "Oh, and I have this other problem. I'm bleeding from my ass" (or chest pain, or shortness of breath, or whatever). You suddenly are no longer my friend. Thanks for putting me twenty minutes behind in one fell swoop. Ugh. There goes my lunch break. Now I'm going to be hungry and subsequently pissed off the rest of the day.

The neighbor who knows everything: we all have one. We all know that one guy who knows someone who had something just like this, and they ended up doing something heroic to him, and now he's doing great (or he died, whichever way you want to go with this). Unless your neighbor is a physician, I'm probably only going to half listen. I'm not saying that the neighbor isn't right, because many times they are, but everyone is different, and many things present the same, so I will evaluate you in a way that is appropriate for you regardless of what your neighbor says. I will always listen, but I may not always agree.

The relative who is a health care professional: is a variation of the know-it-all neighbor. I usually take relatives who work in the field a little more seriously. First of all, depending on who they are, they are usually closer to correct. Even if they are not correct, I will take the necessary steps to rule out what he or she is suggesting. I'm going to have to justify my decision to disagree with them more times than not anyway. Additionally, they have the luxury of spending countless hours researching a problem or chief complaint, so by the time they come in to see me they have a pretty decent idea of what needs to be done. That's a big chunk of my mental energy.

The "what the hell does that have to do with anything"?: so let's start talking about your headache, but then all of a sudden we are talking about your cousin who fell off her horse and broke her pelvis. Huh? It's not really important to know that. Please stick to topic, which is you. The exception might be the family history. If something runs prominently in your family, that would be interesting to know, but your neighbors' medical problems don't really need to be discussed.

The smartass: keeps the sarcasm out of the exam room. Believe it or not I do, so there's no reason why you can't either. I do understand that some people get nervous and are anxious when talking to the doctor, but that's no excuse to be an asshole. It's not funny. I don't appreciate it, and it can be bad for your health if I ask a serious question and you pop off with an attitude. I'm there to help you, but it takes two to communicate.

The scaredy cat/stoic: speaking of communicating, you do need to participate in the conversation. Not telling me something because you are afraid that I will tell you something bad is absolutely the wrong thing to do. If you are having chest pain, I really do need to know about it. Your life literally depends on me knowing what is going on with you. My crystal ball is in the shop, and I can't read your mind. If you can't tell me, then tell someone else and bring him or her in with you. It's not ideal, but it's better than nothing.

The overbearing spouse: this isn't the same as the spouse who has come in to help with the history or to be nosey. I can deal with that. This is the obnoxious version. No one wins with this one. I can't get a history half the time because the wife is sitting in the corner demanding that something be done right now when I'm just trying to figure out why you are even in my exam room. Tell him or her to be quiet for a minute and let me figure out what it is that you have and what we are going to do first. Then we can talk and address concerns. The other scenario is the angry phone call thirty minutes after the appointment demanding to know what we talked about and why some problem or the other that I wasn't even aware of was not addressed. Again, there's no crystal ball. You must communicate with me. I have actually dismissed patients from my practice because the spouse or family member was so difficult. I guarantee if your son calls my office and spews obscenities at my staff, or me, I will dismiss you. At that point, I have lost the ability to be objective, and any further interaction with you would not be in your best interest. From then on I am just trying to avoid interacting with you. No one likes being cursed at, doctors included. Well, maybe nurses do. Just kidding, geeze.

The complaint hoarder/hypochondriac: bring a list. More importantly, bring a list and let me read it. That saves us a lot of time and trouble. I can typically address all your hypochondriacal problems if you write it down and bring it in for me to read. The exception to this is the fellow who is trying to get five or six office visits out of single co-pay. That doesn't work very well. I can't biopsy your suspicious looking lesion, talk about why you get up every thirty minutes at night to take a pee, check your blood pressure, fix your shoulder, treat your jock itch, and talk about routine health maintenance in one ten-minute appointment. You need a full physical, and we need to systematically approach your problems. Sorry, it's going to take more than one appointment. Don't get all put out.

Dr. Google: the problem with Dr. Google isn't the vast amount of knowledge out there on the Internet, it's the fact that there's no perspective placed on that vast amount of knowledge. Give me a list of vague symptoms, such as fatigue, difficulty sleeping, muscles aches, and I can give you any number of conditions that have these as symptoms. Probably dozens if not tens of dozens of conditions fit this bill. I will frequently see the computer print-out of the disease that the patient has convinced herself that she has after surfing the web. In my practice the vast majority of the time this is the wrong diagnosis, and I spend the rest of the office visit convincing the patient of this. I typically do this in the same fashion as having the family member who works in the medical field. I have to disprove their preconception before they consider what I am proposing.

The texter: in this day and age of electronics no one is safe from the cell phone. An informal observation in my office on a random

Thursday last week showed that just about half of the patients in my exam room were either texting or received a phone call during the office visit. The number one reason for the call was a concerned family member asking how the doctor's visit went and what I said. I say turn off your phone before you come into the exam room so that we aren't interrupted. Most people are usually pretty apologetic, so I can't complain too much. Teenagers, however, often don't even put the phone down long enough to get examined. Come on, kids. Show some respect. Oh, and since I'm being all crotchety, get off my lawn.

The know-it-all: no you aren't, period. Just because you took some prerequisite classes in college or trade school, that doesn't make you an expert. Believe me, medicine is much more complicated than you even realize. I don't pretend to know everything. It's impossible for any one human to know everything about medicine. That's why we have specialties. If you know more than me, feel free to get your medical license and start your own practice. Otherwise, consider that maybe I might actually know what I am talking about.

The waffle: make up your mind already. Do you have chest pain or do you not have chest pain? Are you telling me that you only have chest pain if I promise to not tell you that you need your heart looked at, or do you not really have chest pain? I'm not a mind reader. Do you want me to put you on the ventilator if you stop breathing, or don't you? It's kinda important to know ahead of time.

The weekender: there are two variations on the weekender. The first is the Friday night dump. The hospital is not a babysitting service. I understand that sometimes taking care of an elderly parent with dementia is difficult. I really do understand. That's why there are services that will watch them for a day or two so you can take a break. Dropping them off in my office with the vague story that they are weak and dizzy and are falling more so I will admit them to the hospital for testing is not appropriate.

I didn't fall off the naïve truck. I know what you are doing. You're not communicating with me; you're sometimes fabricating and usually embellishing so I will admit them. You know I can't do much from a diagnostic standpoint on a Friday at 4:00 p.m. I will happily work them up as appropriate, but they will go home as soon as the evaluation is complete and I have verified that there is nothing that warrants continued hospitalization. That's usually Saturday morning. I have a lot of pressure from the hospital and insurance companies to get people out of the hospital quickly. I'm not going to lie for you so you can relax and go outlet mall shopping. The other weekender is the fellow who is about half dead and wants me to fix him on a Friday afternoon because he either has a busy weekend planned or is leaving town in the morning. Guess what, you do get admitted and often will stay in the hospital all weekend. If you would have come in earlier in the week, or even earlier in the day, maybe I could have worked you up as an outpatient.

The child herd/uninvolved parent: it's difficult to communicate when little Johnny is tearing apart my exam room. No, those stirrups are not for you. Put them back. Get out of my cabinets. For the love of all things good will you please put down that cell phone and do something with your four kids before I do? I am also a parent. My kids would have been disciplined long ago. Your kids are not attention deficit; they are misbehaved and undisciplined. I have no problem with a child with a legitimate medical condition. Being a brat isn't one of them. Oh, and keep them off of my lawn, since I'm all crotchety today.

To be fair, communication goes both ways. Doctors also fail this one.

The language barrier: patients will often come to me after seeing their specialist for the simple fact that they didn't understand a damn thing he said, and they were hoping that I had his consultation note so I could translate for them. It does help practicing medicine where I grew up since I speak the accent. Sometimes though I also have the same problem with other physicians, especially in the middle of the night when the ER physician who "ain't from around here" is presenting a patient to me for admission to the hospital. I understand that most physicians are not born and raised in cornbread country, but it still affects communication.

The double booker/rusher: time is precious, but that doesn't give the doctor the right to intentionally double book patients. That's just rude. No one likes to wait for three hours to be seen and then only be seen for three or four minutes. I do understand that there are a lot of people who need to be seen. I could work steadily twenty-four hours a day if I chose to. The point isn't to see as many people as possible. It's difficult to be thorough and too easy to miss something that way.

The obsessed: we all have topics that we find interesting. As physicians, we sometimes get too interested to the point of obsession. Being focused is part of the job description. Unfortunately this obsession could be a disease state, a treatment plan, or some aspect of medicine that has nothing to do with why you are even here. If you come in for a cough and leave with labs for cholesterol and a colonoscopy, I may not be doing you any favors. On the other hand, one could make an argument that it's good comprehensive medicine. However, if I can't hear what you are telling me because I am obsessed with what your cholesterol was last year, for example, then communication breaks down.

The distracted: it seems pretty obvious that if I am worried about what my teenage daughter is doing after school or how my ex-wife is going to piss me off this week, I'm not paying enough attention to you. I try to keep that out of the exam room.

The interrupted: doctors have cell phones too, and ours sometimes ring. We get phone calls that we have to take, and emergencies pop up. They are sometimes unavoidable, but they all interrupt the flow of information.

Believe it or not, doctors can be judgmental and abrasive. In my opinion, there's no reason for that. We are in the service industry and need to understand that we are here to help. Yes, you are overweight and don't exercise and have bad habits that will eventually kill you. That doesn't mean I have to be obnoxious when I tell you about it.

The know-it-all: if I think I know everything before you even finish talking then my hubris won't allow me to listen to what you are telling me. I think I already know the answer. That's rather dangerous in my opinion. If I'm not listening to you, then I am failing you.

The tester: there needs to be a balance between clinical suspicion and testing. Running every diagnostic test known to medicine is not only expensive; it can erode the trust between the physician and the patient. I have had patients come to me complaining that the last doctor they saw just ran tests but never told them anything. The patients wondered if the doctor even knew what he was doing.

The denier: it's all in your head. Unfortunately, sometimes it really is, but not as often as some think. I will give the benefit of the doubt. This is a diagnosis of exclusion.

The comedian: yes, we have all seen the movies and watched the television shows. Sometimes it is appropriate to joke with patients, and sometimes it isn't. Off-color humor is not always appreciated. Believe me; I am acutely aware of this one. We as physicians need to understand when it is appropriate and when it is not.

Patient presents for an annual physical examination:

Me: "Hi, how are you doing. What can I do for you?"

Patient: "I'm here for my physical." (Hope that's what they say. Sometimes it's, "You're the doctor. You tell me.")

Me: "Ah, so you're here for a tune-up? Check under the hood, kick the tires, check the oil?"

Patient: "Is that supposed to be funny?"

Me: "Up until now it was hilarious."

The creeper: just as I appreciate you not pawing all over me, so I should return the favor. In my town there is one physician who has the reputation of being just a bit too touchy feely, or significantly too touchy feely depending on who you talk to. It is a small town after all, and everyone hears the rumors. Clearly if you are concerned about Dr. Feelgood feeling you up, you may be less than confident in your physician.

# Home Life

It was my first semester of my first year of medical school. I was supposed to get married the summer between college and medical school, but due to scheduling issues that didn't happen until September, I was about six weeks into school, which was about the time we took our first round of tests. I got married on a Saturday and took my first anatomy exam the following Monday. Needless to say, my score on that test wasn't stellar. Following that test I had this conversation with my Anatomy professor:

Professor: "What happened?"

Me: "That was nothing like I expected."

Professor: "Why didn't you study more?"

Me: "I got married Saturday."

Professor: "Ah, so you were thinking with the little head and not the big head?"

Me: "Um, no, I got married."

Professor: "Well, obviously you weren't thinking."

Me, thinking to myself: *Geeze, you're an asshole. I still have post-traumatic stress disorder. I'm about to jump up and kick your ass.*

Me, actually talking: "I will work harder."

Professor: "You need to understand what it means to be a doctor. Medicine is a jealous mistress. She doesn't like you thinking about anything but her. You're going to have to learn to deal with that."

Me, thinking: *You're still an ass.*

Me, talking: "Yes, sir."

To really do this job properly, the lines between profession and personal life must be blurred. I wish people only became sick between 9:00 a.m. and 5:00 p.m. Monday through Friday, and babies could be born on a schedule. The unfortunate part is that neither do.

Oh sure, some physicians work on shift. ER physicians and urgent care centers are classic examples. They also classically don't do any significant follow up and are not responsible to or for specific individual patients. My patients are my responsibility. That means that either I or one of my partners are available twenty-four hours a day. That's difficult on a family and marriage.

I don't know how many school events I have missed due to patient obligations, dozens I'm sure. I don't plan my week more than two hours in advance, because I can't. I don't know how my children are doing in school, because they are usually in bed before I get home from work, and the kids understand that Daddy doesn't like taking vacations because when he does one of his patients usually dies because they won't see anyone else.

My wife is also now my ex-wife, in part because my profession sometimes has no choice but to take precedence.

Notice that this is a short chapter. Medicine is a jealous mistress.

# Fraud and You

Unfortunately, one's ability to retain knowledge and take a test does not correlate to higher levels of morality. As with any profession, there are those who are honest and those who are less so. Medical fraud is unfortunately very real—not only by physicians, but the entire health care industry.

No one knows exactly how much health care fraud costs this country, but the Department of Health and Human Services (HHS) estimates it to be in the billions of dollars each year.[81] Fraud can be demonstrated many ways, such as payment for nonexistent goods or services, unnecessary medical services, claims with insufficient documentation, and payment for ineligible patients and to ineligible providers are some examples. Other examples include misrepresenting services, altering claim forms for higher payments, and falsification of medical record documents. There are many real life examples.

In Texas, a supplier of durable medical equipment was found guilty of five counts of health care fraud due to submission of false claims to Medicare. Raritan Bay Medical Center agreed to pay the government 7.5 million dollars to settle allegations that it defrauded the Medicare program, purposely inflating charges for inpatient and outpatient care. AmeriGroup Illinois, Inc., fraudulently skewed enrolment into the Medicaid HMO program by refusing to register pregnant women and discouraging registration for individuals with pre-existing conditions. In Florida, a dermatologist was sentenced to twenty-two years in prison, paid 3.7 million dollars in restitution, and paid a 25,000 dollar fine for performing 3,086 medically unnecessary surgeries on 865 Medicare beneficiaries.[82] The US Department of Health and Human Services Office of the Inspector General (OIG) also found in an audit that providers in eight out of ten states received approximately 27.3 million dollars in Medicaid overpayments for services claimed after beneficiaries' deaths.[83]

So, then, how do we combat fraud, waste, and abuse in the health care industry? Data modelling and mining techniques is perhaps the most valuable tool for detecting fraud and abuse.[84] Automated data mining technologies allow the government and other institutions to gain valuable insights and to detect patterns within data without predetermined bias. Statistical algorithms can be used to identify general trends or patterns of suspicious transactions in health care data. This takes me to the requirement for electronic health records. Once again HIPPA established rules for access, authentications, storage, auditing, and transmittal of electronic medical records. This was followed closely by the 2009 HITECH Act, which put teeth on the HIPPA requirements for electronic medical records.[85] As per usual, these teeth are financial. Physicians who adopt electronic medical records (EMR) systems prior to 2015 will receive incentive payments, but those who do not adopt an EHR by 2015 will be penalized 1 percent of Medicare payments, increasing to 3 percent over three years.[86] My office was one of the first private practices in my state to adopt and qualify for a Meaningful Use Incentive Payment. It was not at all easy or simple.

There are three stages required to meet Meaningful Use.[87] Currently only the first stage is well defined. For a private practice, the first stage contains twenty-five measures. These objectives have been divided into a core set and optional menu set.

Physicians must meet all objectives/measures in the core set plus five of ten optional items.

Core requirements:

1. Use computerized order entry for medication orders.
2. Implement drug-drug, drug-allergy checks.
3. Generate and transmit permissible prescriptions electronically.
4. Record demographics.
5. Maintain an up-to-date problem list of current and active diagnoses.
6. Maintain active medication list.
7. Maintain active medication allergy list.
8. Record and chart changes in vital signs.
9. Record smoking status for patients thirteen years old or older.
10. Implement one clinical decision support rule.
11. Report ambulatory quality measures to CMS or the States.
12. Provide patients with an electronic copy of their health information upon request.
13. Provide clinical summaries to patients for each office visit.
14. Capability to exchange key clinical information electronically among providers and patient authorized entities.
15. Protect electronic health information (privacy and security).

Optional Requirements:

1. Implement drug-formulary checks.
2. Incorporate clinical lab-test results into certified EHR as structured data.

3. Generate lists of patients by specific conditions to use for quality improvement, reduction of disparities, research, and outreach.

4. Send reminders to patients per patient preference for preventive/follow-up care.

5. Provide patients with timely electronic access to their health information (including lab results, problem list, medication lists, allergies).

6. Use certified EHR to identify patient-specific education resources and provide to patient if appropriate.

7. Perform medication reconciliation as relevant.

8. Provide summary care record for transitions in care or referrals.

9. Capability to submit electronic data to immunization registries and actual submission.

10. Capability to provide electronic syndromic surveillance data to public health agencies and actual transmission.

To receive this "incentive" money (or to not be penalized down the road), CMS requires participants in the Medicare EHR Incentive Program to "attest" that during a ninety-day reporting period, they used a certified EHR and met stage one criteria for Meaningful Use objectives and clinical quality measures. The requirements above, although on the surface do not sound unreasonable, the satisfactory reporting of these requirements is onerous and laborious, even through "attestation" (also called the "pinky promise" or "cross my heart I am telling the truth" method). Unfortunately, in our practice it required hiring another staff member at significant cost whose sole job is to manage, track, and verify compliance with Meaningful Use. Future stages will require the demonstration of compliance through appropriate reporting systems, which are currently under development and testing. The law in this instance is ahead of the current technology. EMR companies have been scrambling to create software and interfaces that can mine data, interact with other systems, and report in a manner that meets the requirements of Meaningful Use. Of course for every upgrade, system change, or interface, there is a fee.

The government predicts that the startup of an EMR system will cost roughly 16,000 to 36,000 dollars per physician, and over time increased revenue from lost charges and under-coding will more than make up for the initial startup cost.[88] In a private practice, there isn't extra cash sitting around. In my office we would sit at the table every month and determine how we were going to pay our staff their salary without borrowing money to do it. This was not due to a mismanaged office; it was due to zero profit margins. If Medicare withheld payment for a week or a month due to a system upgrade, or a private insurance decided this week it wasn't going to process claims appropriately, we would have to often borrow against a line of credit to pay our employees until the money came in. That is unfortunately not a sustainable business model. I assure you also, we as physicians and business owners were not pillaging the system. For family practice, the slowest physician in my office worked at the eightieth percentile of productivity and generated revenue equal to or above that. Most of us worked at greater than the ninetieth percentile as determined by MGMA (Medical Group Management Association). The MGMA collects, processes, and then disseminates data, which hospitals and private practices then use to compare themselves to other practices nationally or regionally. Our personal income was in the thirtieth percentile. The remaining revenue went to the 72 percent overhead that we carried. Billing and collecting was streamlined. Our days in AR (accounts receivable, money billed but waiting to be collected) were sixteen days on average. An "excellent" AR is thirty days. We billed the day of service and aggressively tracked and followed up on claims sent to the insurance companies. There was no room for improvement.

I do not know where the government's 32,000 dollars startup cost number quoted comes from, but I suspect that possibly the EMR companies trying to sell the systems. That is about what the software alone costs. Add on the hardware requirements, and I guarantee the startup cost and ongoing maintenance cost is significantly more than that.[89] In addition to having to meet the requirements for Meaningful Use, which required us to hire a dedicated staff member, the startup of our EMR system cost about a quarter million for the entire office, which was close to fifty thousand dollars per physician. This included servers, computers for us and all our staff, new diagnostic equipment that interfaces with our EMR, and fiber optic Internet connection with numerous wireless access points.

In addition to startup cost, we are required through necessity to maintain a pricey support contract through the various vendors. Add the now necessary full time information technology (IT) specialist to keep the hardware, software, and interfaces operational. To meet Meaningful Use, there must be an exchange of information. Electronic prescribing, lab orders, and transmission to the state health department require software interfaces. For every required interface, such as lab interface, patient portal interface, medical equipment interface, hospital interface, and electronic prescribing, we are charged an initial costly startup fee as well as an ongoing maintenance fee that must continue to be paid to meet the requirements set forth in 2009 HITECH and HIPPA.

In my practice with efficient coding and billing, we saw only about a 5 percent increase in gross revenue. This was attributed to capturing missed charges, such as ancillary testing that we failed to bill for, and a small amount of under-coding that we now had the documentation to demonstrate the correct billing level.

I do not need a computer to talk to a patient, take a history, perform an examination, and treat. The benefit that I derive from all this is the luxury of not getting financially penalized or jailed for medical fraud.

This brings me back to HIPPA. Efforts to combat fraud were consolidated and strengthened under Public Law 104-191, the Health Insurance Portability and Accountability Act of 1996 (HIPAA).[90] The Act established a comprehensive program to combat fraud committed against all health plans, both public and private. This enhanced the ability of the federal government to recoup inappropriate health care spending. One method by which this occurs is by allowing the Department of Health and Human Services (HHS) to enter into contracts with private entities to review and audit activities where Medicare provides coverage. These contracts will allow private organizations to review health care professionals and others providing services, audit cost reports, determine whether a Medicare payment should have been made, and initiate recovery of Medicare payments that should not have been made.

Additionally, funding was increased, which almost doubled the number of HHS OIG (Office of the Inspector General) auditors and investigators in addition to expanding the Federal Bureau of Investigation's (FBI) ability to investigate health care fraud. This additional funding also established a monetary reward program to encourage Medicare beneficiaries to report virtually anything they believe to be questionable behavior. The American Medical Association warns that anyone submitting a claim for payment must be alert to the potential for liability stemming from an inappropriately submitted claim. In paying a claim, the federal government has the authority to investigate the properness of the claim. If an investigation finds fault with a claim, the government has the authority to impose either criminal or civil sanctions (monetary fines and exclusion from the Medicare and Medicaid programs) against the individual or entity claiming a right to payment, depending on the nature of the inappropriate conduct. If there is a determination that even a single claim was submitted fraudulently, sanctions may include imprisonment for up to five years a fine of up 250,000 dollars per claim, and exclusion from participation in the Medicare and Medicaid programs.[91]

Giving more authority to HIPPA are provisions found in the Affordable Care Act, which went into effect May 2010. This Act increases the federal sentencing guidelines for health care fraud offenses by 20 to 50 percent for certain crimes and establishes penalties for obstructing a fraud investigation or audit, making it easier for the government to recapture any inappropriately distributed funds. It allows for better communication and coordination between law enforcement amongst states through increased coordination, intelligence sharing, and training among investigators, agents, prosecutors, analysts, and policymakers.[92]

In my average day I am audited routinely. My clinical judgments and treatments are peer reviewed. My office notes are audited for completeness and appropriateness by my "boss," a director with a master's degree in health care administration, which bases an annual financial incentive that I may or may not receive on my ability to appropriately chart. I also routinely undergo HEDIS (Health care Effectiveness Data and Information Set) audits, which are audits to verify that I am following the standard of care and appropriately documenting. HEDIS is a tool used by more than 90 percent of America's health plans to measure performance that allows a reliable comparison of the performance of health care plans/providers. HEDIS altogether consists of seventy-six measures across five domains of care. Some common benchmarks include appropriate asthma medication use (by appropriate they mean following the algorithm), breast cancer screening, blood pressure control, immunization status, and diabetes care.[93]

I am audited by my billing department for appropriate billing and use of billing modifiers. A billing modifier is a number or letter combination that is attached to a bill sent to the insurance company for payment. There are numerous modifiers, and the Medicare billing modifier guide is a mere fifty-two pages. If I perform a procedure as well and have an office visit, I must attach a -25 modifier to the office visit billing code, or the claim will be rejected or not paid. If I give more than one unit of a medication, then I must add a numerical modifier such as -4 for four units. If I give an immunization, then I must add an immunization procedure code, unless of course there are two immunizations, then I use the single and the multiple code. I must use a different code on a Medicare patient than a private insurance patient. If I perform a procedure in the period immediately after a surgery that is unrelated to the surgery, then I must add a different modifier, and so on.

There are a significant number of modifiers, and the list is a moving target, changing from year to year. Our billing staff is specifically trained in knowing these and go to frequent training seminars to keep current on the upcoming changes. They then come back and try to teach me the proper use of these modifiers. In addition to understanding medicine, I am also expected to have a good grasp of the current billing regulations. Appropriate billing refers to knowing what billing level is appropriate to the visit.

In the golden age, office visits were billed pretty standard across the board. A person went to the doctor and was charged a flat fee for services. At some point before my time this changed to a tiered system. Office visit charges became graded, so that it may be simple, moderate complexity, or high complexity. Whether the patient had been seen in the office in the last two years also affects how much the office visit is billed. Whether the visit is from a primary care physician or a specialist, whether it is a consultation, and whether it is a visit for preventative service also plays a role in the level of billing and the code attached to the billing requisition.

The level of the visit is determined less by what I physically do in the exam room, but more by the level of detail and the documentation of the visit. The level of complexity of the history, the detail of the physical examination, and the risk and medical decision making involved all are taken into account to determine the level of the visit. This is vitally important. Not only does it determine how much I have to bill you, failure to do so can result in financial and criminal penalties. The CMS basic guide is an eighty-nine-page document, which directly states the following:

> Billing Medicare requires the selection of a Current Procedural Terminology (CPT) code that best represents the patient type, the setting of service, and the Evaluation and Management (E&M) level. For purposes of billing for E/M services, patients are identified as either new or established, depending on previous encounters with the provider. The setting can be an office or other outpatient setting; hospital inpatient, emergency department, and nursing facility.
>
> The code sets used to bill for E/M services are organized into various categories and levels. In general, the more complex the visit, the higher the level of code the physician may bill within the appropriate category. In order to bill any code, the services furnished must meet the definition of the code. It is the physician's responsibility to ensure that the codes selected reflect the services furnished.
>
> There are three key components when selecting the appropriate level of E/M service provided: history, examination, and medical decision-making.

As the rest of this summary is quite dry and incredibly boring, it can be found in Appendix A. If you want to know why I charged you 117 dollars for that office visit, please refer there first.

This, of course, is only the basic overview. Once this is understood, there are rules, which vary depending on the situation. This is only one of the things I am thinking about in the exam room as we discuss your medical condition. From a purely administrative standpoint, I must be sure to document everything appropriately.

If I do not it could end poorly for me. My current employer audits my notes, and I am financially penalized for both under-coding an encounter or the worse of the two, over-coding an encounter. We fear the over-code.

This brings me to the RAC ("rack") audit. The threat of a RAC audit is told to young health care professionals late at night around the heart monitors and IV pumps to scare them. It is the Boogey monster of audits. In an effort to expand overpayment recovery efforts, CMS through authority created by the Tax Relief and Health Care Act of 2006, has teamed up with private organizations to create the Recovery Audit Contractor (RAC) program, which is expected to recover 2.1 billion dollars in Medicare overpayments in the first five years. In a nutshell, the RAC program is a fee-for-service program in which an independent contractor will audit medical records, looking for overpayments. If overpayments are found, the institution, whether it is a large organization such as a health care conglomerate or a single physician office, will repay the overpayment to the RAC contractor. The contractor will keep a percentage of the recovered amount and return the rest to the insurance institution, usually CMS.[94, 95] In theory this sounds like a good idea, but here is where the horror starts.

My office was independent, and even with multiple providers and as lean an operation as physically possible, it would not have survived a RAC audit if any significant overpayment were found. There is no financial margin in a primary care office. It would have been a business death sentence, one that would have not been recoverable.

One of the fears of a billing audit is that to a certain extent some of the coding is subjective. Even if the documentation provided supports the level of billing, there is, in certain circumstances, an instance where the "spirit" of the encounter may be one billing level when in fact the documentation supports another.[96] A good example is the documentation generated by an electronic medical record system. Because an electronic record keeps everything (unless, like in my case, the servers fail and I lose three days of patient encounters), it will put a significant amount of information in the clinical note. Many electronic medical records (EMRs) have automatic calculators, which will determine the level of billing based upon the amount of documentation provided.

Unfortunately, this is not a foolproof method of billing. Take the example of the common cold. A patient presents to my office with a cold. I evaluate him and determine that he indeed has a cold. I reassure him, we discuss chicken soup, and he goes home. Since the EMR system imported his entire past medical history into the note, which may or may not necessarily be relevant in this particular case, the calculator may actually code this visit as a moderate complexity visit when in reality it was a lower-level visit as the risk was low, and no medications were prescribed. A RAC audit may find this to be a low-level visit despite the documentation, and the provider will be penalized. RAC audits do not pay providers and institutions if under-coding takes place, so there is a bit of a double standard here as well. There is no element of fairness. I can either code appropriately with the fear of over-coding or routinely under-code and eventually go bankrupt.

The only two outcomes if an audit takes place is complete disruption of workflow during the audit with zero benefit, or a complete disruption of workflow with a financial or possible criminal penalty. Additionally, since the contracted "bounty hunters" work off of a percentage of claims found, I cannot imagine an audit that would be in any way objective. The coder, like human nature dictates, will look out for his or her best interests. I'm sure they have bills to pay also. Their incentive is to penalize so that they recover a larger amount. Given the somewhat subjective nature of coding, this gives me pause as a shudder of apprehension passes through.

Another way CMS attempts to curb fraud is through closer regulations of such things as home health services and DME, or durable medical equipment. Durable medical equipment is basically any equipment that can be reused, hence durable. Crutches, walkers, wheelchairs, and oxygen equipment are all examples of durable medical equipment.

In 2010 CMS stated that, under the Affordable Care Act, physicians must actually see the patient face to face and document the need for DME as well as home health and hospice services. Although this makes life slightly more complicated from my standpoint, I can see how it will be beneficial in cost containment. I am now obligated to have an appointment specifically addressing the issue of home health, hospice, or equipment. Previously, in some instances home health services and equipment were ordered with minimal or no documentation from the physician, such as when the patient was discharged from the hospital or rehabilitation facility. In these instances, the patient would occasionally receive services or equipment that may not be medically necessary. There was little regulation from a clinical standpoint as it is impossible for a physician or even an entire health care team to know what is happening to every patient all the time, especially if the patient is at another health care facility, such as a hospital.

The Act also tightened enrollment and screening and instituted competitive bidding for companies who participate in Medicare. Competitive bidding does have the drawback that a patient may not have the luxury of being able to have all home equipment services provided by "one stop shop," requiring them to obtain equipment from whichever vendor can supply the equipment at the lowest cost.[97]

# Herding Cats

"I have eight bosses, Bob."

"Pardon me?"

"Eight Bosses."

"Eight?"

"Eight, Bob! That means that when I screw something up, I have to hear eight different people tell me about it."

—Office Space, 1999

Controlling doctors is like herding cats. In theory, it's possible, but extremely difficult. I am an independent thinker. I have to be. I have to feel confident in my ability to make decisions and stand by that decision, even if it's unpopular. Tragically, it appears the only carrot that physicians classically respond consistently to is monetary.[98] Apparently the best way to influence the behavior of a physician is attach a financial incentive or penalty to it. If the 2009 HITECH Act, which strengthens the civil and criminal enforcement of the HIPAA rules, is any indication, CMS is very aware of this.[99] I personally find this disheartening on several levels. First is the integrity factor. As a professional and health care provider, I do try to do the right thing every time. To think that there has to be a financial carrot and/or stick (to a maximum penalty of 1.5 million dollars) to do what I would hope is the right thing to begin with saddens me.

Regardless, on any given day a number of external forces will pressure me to practice medicine in one manner or the other. Often this is contrary to what I believe is in the best interest of the patient and the standard of medical care. In the days before I started swinging a stethoscope as a civilian, often referred by the old timers as the "golden age" of medicine, stories are told that the only influences a physician had to deal with was a pharmaceutical representative in an alluring business suit trying to direct prescribing practices. I have been told by some of my elders that the pharmaceutical representatives would bring in lunch, have educational dinners, pass out freebies such as office supplies and gadgets, and even sponsor things like educational seminars to vacation-like locales. Of course, that was before my time.

As a military physician we were not allowed, through federal mandates, to receive gifts from sales representatives, and in 2009 PhRMA, the Pharmaceutical Research and Manufacturers of America, which represents research-based pharmaceutical and biotechnology companies, adopted an updated and enhanced voluntary Code on relationships with US health care professionals.[100] This builds upon the standards and principles set forth in its predecessor, the PhRMA Code on Interactions with Health Care Professionals that took effect on July 1, 2002. Like the 2002 edition, which significantly restricted the activities of the pharmaceutical representatives, the 2009 code addressed how pharmacy reps interacted with physicians with respect to marketed products and related activities. It prohibited small gifts and reminder items such as pens, notepads, staplers, and clipboards, as well as prohibited company sales representatives from providing restaurant meals to health care professionals outside their offices.[101, 102] I occasionally see the remains of these bygone times with an old anatomic model here or a refrigerator magnet there.

Today pressures to influence my medical decisions come from other third party entities.

A pharmacy refused to fill a medication because a medication adverse effect, in this case nausea or stomach upset, was noted in the patient's record on file at the pharmacy. Adverse effects, such as stomach upset, are quite common in certain classes of medications. These are not allergies, only unfortunate and expected effects of the medication. Again, as a physician, I must weigh the risks of the medication versus the benefits of the medication. In this particular instance the prescription written was for a medication of a similar class as the medication that caused the adverse effect. It was not the same class. The risk for adverse effect was no higher or lower than any other medication on any other patient.

An insurance company refused to pay for a medication unless the patient had an unnecessary diagnostic test performed. I can only guess that the company wished to prove or disprove the diagnosis for which this particular medication was ordered. However, in this particular case the patient had a medical condition in which this medication, although not FDA approved, would benefit the patient greatly. Medications are often used for many reasons, some of which are not necessarily approved through the FDA. This "off-label" use is very common. I use every tool in my proverbial toolbox. Sometimes I use a wrench as a hammer, so to speak. To obtain FDA approval for all uses for a medication is time consuming and expensive. Therefore, not all medications have FDA approval for all indications with which the medication works.

A nutritionist requested labs. Upon evaluation, it was determined that the patient had relevant lab work less than a month prior and was not due for any additional labs. I respectfully declined, but was inundated with repeated requests.

A pharmacist review at the nursing home in which I have patients and am medical director requested that I check routine labs, adjust medication dose, and change medications from one to

another despite maximal medical management and patient sta-
bility. This is every day. Some of these requests are mandated by
the government in the form of CMS guidelines, such as those
requiring dosage adjustments of psychotropic medications and
antipsychotics. These are typically grounded in good medicine,
and although I take offence at adjusting medications on patients
who are doing well on the meds they have been on sometimes
for years, I do understand the rationale and usually begrudgingly
comply. Sometimes experience with the patient tells me that a
medication adjustment is not at all indicated due to the stabil-
ity, or relative instability, of the patient. Not all people fit into
an algorithm.

Some of these requests are due to the cost of the medication. Long-term care facilities work closely with pharmacists to
identify less expensive alternatives to more costly medications to
help with cost containment. Although this is admirable, not all
medications of the same class work similarly.

A prime and relatively elementary example is the use of cholesterol lowering medications called statins. They are all of the
same class, but each one works very differently. It is well known
that lowering cholesterol reduces risk for heart attacks and other
cardiovascular events, but it's not that simple. Although lowering
LDL (Low Density Lipoprotein, one component of total cholesterol) is almost always the goal of therapy, it's not the only
target. Secondary targets, notably triglycerides and high-den-
sity lipoproteins (HDL), need to be considered in higher risk
patients.[103] In addition, each cholesterol medicine works somewhat differently.

All statins can reduce LDL by up to 35 percent. However,
the following medications can reduce LDL by up to 50 percent:
atorvastatin (20 mg or higher dose), lovastatin (80 mg or higher),
rosuvastatin (10 mg or higher), simvastatin (20 mg or higher),
niacin plus lovastatin (1000/40 or higher), and ezetimibe plus
simvastatin (10/20 mg). In studies directly comparing statins at

the highest doses, atorvastatin (80 mg) lowered LDL-c more than simvastatin (80 mg) but resulted in more adverse events, while rosuvastatin (40 mg) was superior to atorvastatin (80 mg) in reducing LDL levels and resulted in a similar frequency of adverse events. But that's not all we look at. We also take into consideration HDL, or good cholesterol. Some studies found that simvastatin and rosuvastatin were superior to atorvastatin in increasing HDL. Niacin also works well to raise HDL, but due to the side effect of flushing often described as "hot flashes," it is not well tolerated by many. Additionally, Even if LDL cholesterol is optimal, additive treatment with niacin and fibrates should be considered for patients with diabetes or metabolic syndrome, if triglycerides are high, HDL is low, or both. Often statins work preferentially better on other components of the lipid panel such as the triglycerides, which, by sticking to a slightly more costly medication, eliminates the need for an additional lipid lowering medication and the resultant adverse effects, medication interactions, and polypharmacy.[104]

So basically, it's not as simple as saying that since this medication is in the same class, it must work the same as another medication in the same class. But since a therapeutic interchange will save the long-term care facility twenty bucks or so annually, the request winds up on my desk, repeatedly and persistently if I deny it. Which brings me to a decision: Do I continue to disagree and expect to get a medication interchange request weekly, or do I give in and change the medication, which results in suboptimal management of the patient's medical condition?

This brings me to the therapeutic interchange. State pharmacy laws allow, in certain circumstances, a pharmacist to substitute a product from the same class of drug, even though they are not therapeutically equivalent.[105] An example would be one statin for another or one blood pressure medication of a particular class with an entirely different medication in the same class. The laws covering therapeutic interchange vary widely from state to state.

Many managed care plans have formularies that allow therapeutic interchange. The placement of a patient on a medication that is not on the insurance or institution's preferred medication list is, from my standpoint, quite difficult and time consuming even though it may be in the best interest of the patient. Sometimes a patient cannot tolerate one medication in a class due to side effects but can tolerate another. I have an employee who spends her entire day dedicated to addressing issues like this.

I hear stories about legal ramifications of therapeutic interchange. The loss of control when formulary management determines drug choice has led to speculation that potential serious litigation could arise from professional activities associated with this practice. Despite this concern, there have been no successful lawsuits involving therapeutic interchange documented. However, that does not mean that there haven't been lawsuits. That's an important difference, especially in a small town.

In order for the plaintiff to succeed in a negligence action, four basic components must be established: (1) that the health care facility or practitioner owed the patient a duty to provide an accepted standard of care; (2) that the health care system breached that duty; (3) that the breach of duty resulted in injury to the patient; and (4) that the patient sustained legally recognized damages as a result.[106] The vast majority of medical negligence and malpractice cases is settled out of court and never become public record. However, if Betty, who we all remember is a gossip, gets wind of it, it can still be devastating.

Sometimes an insurance company flat refuses to cover a medication or even an entire class of medication. Due to cost, this basically eliminates that medication from my available options even though it may be the best choice for the patient. I am still legally responsible for the care of the patient. If Mrs. Jones cannot afford her inhaler for her asthma, then she cannot afford her inhaler, and she goes without. Again, who is de facto practicing medicine? Depending on the situation I sometimes can find a similar substitute, especially if I use medications off-label, but it is not always ideal. Sometimes it feels as though I am patching people up with duct tape and chewing gum. Does this "creative pharmacology" constitute a failure to provide an accepted standard of care and a breach of duty? Unfortunately, the brunt of the liability does not rest with the insurance company who denied coverage, but with me.

Other providers also try to influence my medical decisions. I received a call from a nurse practitioner requesting that a long-standing patient of mine be referred to a neurologist. He was wishing to disqualify this patient from obtaining a commercial driver's license. Upon speaking to him, he stated that based upon my notes, the patient had suffered a cerebrovascular accident and was therefore disqualified for at least a year and required a neurologist evaluation. In my clinical notes it was clearly stated that patient suffered from hypertension and, at onset of this hypertension, suffered what is called a hypertensive urgency and after appropriate medical management was returned to normal. The symptoms are, on the surface, similar to a neurologic event. Physiologically they are very different. Do we know what we don't know?

What does it mean to practice medicine? Again, it is the evaluation and management of a patient by a physician. Today I saw a patient who presented to my office with a stack of papers. In this stack were results of a large panel of blood tests, X-rays, and biometric testing such as body mass index, height, weight, waist circumference, etc. His reason for the visit was to discuss these findings. I asked him who ordered these tests and what follow-up from these tests did he receive. He stated that, through his employer, his insurance carrier runs batteries of tests on him annually. I can only presume without physician supervision, hence his visit to my office. In this patient's particular case, the laboratory testing performed on him was, for the most part, not appropriate for any screening and were also essentially normal.

I discussed the findings, discussed what I would have looked for and why, and sent him on his merry way. He did have some tests results that, although not in the normal range by lab standards, were not clinically significant. I discussed these with him. Whoever ordered the blood tests did not or could not interpret his laboratory findings.

In Indiana, my home state, practicing medicine is strictly defined under IC 25-22.5-1-1.1:

Definitions

Sec. 1.1. As used in this article:

(a) "Practice of medicine or osteopathic medicine" means any one (1) or a combination of the following:

(1) Holding oneself out to the public as being engaged in:

(A) the diagnosis, treatment, correction, or prevention of any disease, ailment, defect, injury, infirmity, deformity, pain, or other condition of human beings;

(B) the suggestion, recommendation, or prescription or administration of any form of treatment, without limitation;

(C) the performing of any kind of surgical operation upon a human being, including tattooing, except for tattooing (as defined in IC 35-42-2-7), in which human tissue is cut, burned, or vaporized by the use of any mechanical means, laser, or ionizing radiation, or the penetration of the skin or body orifice by any means, for the intended palliation, relief, or cure; or

(D) the prevention of any physical, mental, or functional ailment or defect of any person.

(2) The maintenance of an office or a place of business for the reception, examination, or treatment of persons suffering from disease, ailment, defect, injury, infirmity, deformity, pain, or other conditions of body or mind.

(3) Attaching the designation "doctor of medicine", "M.D.", "doctor of osteopathy", "D.O.", "osteopathic medical physician", "physician", "surgeon", or "physician and surgeon", either alone or in connection with other words, or any other words or abbreviations to a name, indicating or inducing others to believe that the person is engaged in the practice of medicine or osteopathic medicine (as defined in this section).

(4) Providing diagnostic or treatment services to a person in Indiana when the diagnostic or treatment services:

(A) are transmitted through electronic communications; and

(B) are on a regular, routine, and nonepisodic basis or under an oral or written agreement to regularly provide medical services.

In addition to the exceptions described in section 2 of this chapter, a nonresident physician who is located outside Indiana does not practice medicine or osteopathy in Indiana by providing a second opinion to a licensee or diagnostic or treatment services to a patient in Indiana following medical care originally provided to the patient while outside Indiana.

(b) "Board" refers to the medical licensing board of Indiana.

(c) "Diagnose or diagnosis" means to examine a patient, parts of a patient's body, substances taken or removed from a patient's body, or materials produced by a patient's body to determine the source or nature of a disease or other physical or mental condition, or to hold oneself out or represent that a person is a physician and is so examining a patient. It is not necessary that the examination be made in the presence of the patient; it may be made on information supplied either directly or indirectly by the patient.

(d) "Drug or medicine" means any medicine, compound, or chemical or biological preparation intended for internal or external use of humans, and all substances intended to be used for the diagnosis, cure, mitigation, or prevention of diseases or abnormalities of humans, which are recognized in the latest editions published of the United States Pharmacopoeia or National Formulary, or otherwise established as a drug or medicine.

(e) "Licensee" means any individual holding a valid unlimited license issued by the board under this article.

(f) "Prescribe or prescription" means to direct, order, or designate the use of or manner of using a drug, medicine, or treatment, by spoken or written words or other means.

(g) "Physician" means any person who holds the degree of doctor of medicine or doctor of osteopathy or its equivalent and who holds a valid unlimited license to practice medicine or osteopathic medicine in Indiana.

(h) "Medical school" means a nationally accredited college of medicine or of osteopathic medicine approved by the board.

(i) "Physician assistant" means an individual who:

    (1) is supervised by a physician;

    (2) graduated from a physician assistant program accredited by an accrediting agency (as defined in IC 25-27.5-2-4.5);

    (3) passed the examination administered by the National Commission on Certification of Physician Assistants (NCCPA) and maintains certification; and

    (4) has been licensed by the physician assistant committee under IC 25-27.5.

(j) "Agency" refers to the Indiana professional licensing agency under IC 25-1-5.

As I read the regulation, per IC Section 25-22.5-1-1.1 (c) specifically stating "Diagnose or diagnosis" means to examine a patient, parts of a patient's body, substances taken or removed from a patient's body, or materials produced by a patient's body to determine the source or nature of a disease or other physical or mental condition." Does drawing blood for lab tests constitute examining substances removed from a patient's body to determine nature of a disease, such as high cholesterol? I think it does. By Indiana code, then, it seems to me that insurance companies who routinely draw panels of labs are practicing medicine. Additionally, medicine is also described as "the suggestion, recommendation, or prescription or administration of any form of treatment, without limitation." The dozen or so daily recommendations from pharmacists, dieticians, physical therapists, nurse case managers, and anonymous insurance company employees with a checklist all suggest and recommend treatment. Is that, then, practicing medicine? Is preferentially paying for one service over another, or authorizing payment for services only when certain criteria are met, then practicing medicine?

In my exam room I am the advocate, not only to diagnose and treat, but to do what is in the best interest of the patient. As the boundaries of what is considered practicing medicine blur, I find this task more and more difficult. Do I treat the patient as a human being and an individual, or do I notate the mountain of information required of me and process the patient through the system, performing all required testing and diagnostics as required by law and recommendations by third-party entities? As medicine evolves, more and more I think, maybe I should have been an electrician.

# The Future of Health Care

Medicine is changing rapidly in America. According to the crusty old-timer physicians in my office, medicine has changed more in the first decade of the twenty-first century than it has in the last thirty years combined. For better or worse, there are more changes yet to come.

With the advent of the computer age and the ability to analyze massive amounts of information quickly, the "art" of medicine is rapidly becoming the "science" of medicine. Analyzing research to determine the most appropriate patient treatment methods is not a new idea. Traces of this can be found as far back as ancient Greece; but it was Andreas Vesalius in the 11th Century who marked the beginning of scientific research and observation.[107] By direct observation through dissection he discovered, recorded, and published the facts of human anatomy. However, the systematic assimilation of all available research to create a generally accepted national treatment recommendation is quite new.

As a matter of fact, my daughter is the same age as "modern" medicine. The term "evidence-based medicine," also called "clinical evidence," a systematic approach to analyze published research as the basis of clinical decision making, was first described in the 1990s.[108] Now, two decades later, we are really beginning to implement the consistent use of this scientific method to determine actual patient treatments. More specifically, we are moving away from anecdotal and traditional treatments and toward this evidence-based medicine (EBM). One definition of EBM is "the conscientious, explicit and judicious use of current best evidence in making decisions about the care of individual patients. The practice of evidence-based medicine means integrating individual clinical expertise with the best available external clinical evidence from systematic research."[109]

I would like to discuss this point a little more. It is so very important that we as a society understand what evidence-based medicine is and what it is not. Without this understanding, I feel the profession of medicine is in serious peril. First of all, medicine is not an exact science. It never has been, and it never will be. The reason for this is simple; humans are all made differently; we are not made on an assembly line. We have both genetic and environmental influences that make us who we are, and one-size treatment does not fit all. Given this, we can sometimes generalize treatments that for the most part work for most people. But how do we decide what works and what doesn't work? Simply, it's trial and error. Its trial and error on both a population level as well as on an individual level, as not everyone responds the same to treatment.

The Hippocratic Oath tells us that as physicians, we are charged with teaching future generations. Of course we have anatomy texts and biochemistry texts and any number of books on the basic sciences. How we integrate the basic sciences and turn that knowledge base into the ability to effectively evaluate and manage a patient has been, for the most part, taught by word of mouth. I learned how to treat most conditions in my residency not by reading a book, but by listening to my teachers. They, in turn, learned how to practice medicine by listening to their teachers and by the best teacher of all—experience. The origins of the medical "clinical" textbooks were originally the transcribed lessons learned by our predecessors. Over time, with each subsequent edition, more and more evidence-based treatments are incorporated, but we must understand that its origins are from observation and experimentation.

When I was a kid, I loved going to my grandparents' house outside of Chicago during the summer. More importantly, I loved their basement. My grandfather was a television repairman in the days of vacuum tubes. His garage, therefore, had all sorts of neat gadgets and tools that I enjoyed playing with and imagining what they did. They also had a guest room/den in the basement where I slept when I visited. On their bookcase they had an eclectic collection of reading materials that, as a young teenager, I could submerse myself into while the adults did whatever adults did upstairs. One of the books on the shelf was entitled *A Physician in the House*, copyright 1897.[110] I used to enjoy reading this book, especially as I grew older, eventually went to medical school, and understood what it meant. Another book, *Library of Health*, refuted the work of Pasteur and germ theory. It also talked about treatment options for various disease states with I think I remember having such names as Latin for "that red rash disease" or "that other red rash disease" or "the disease that makes you turn yellow and feel bad."[111] When my grandparents passed, I was fortunate enough to obtain these books. To read this text and compare it to what we know today is wondrous. Modern medicine is only in its infancy. We really have just begun to scratch the surface in regards to medical treatments. and EBM, if properly assimilated, will advance medicine to levels that we can only imagine.

According to their website, the US Preventive Services Task Force (USPSTF) is an independent panel of non-Federal experts in prevention and evidence-based medicine and is composed of primary care providers (such as internists, pediatricians, family physicians, gynecologists/obstetricians, nurses, and health behavior specialists). They conduct scientific evidence reviews of a broad range of clinical preventive health care services (such as screening, counseling, and preventive medications) and develop recommendations for primary care clinicians and health systems.[112] These recommendations are published in the form of "recommendation statements." They strive to make accurate, up-to-date, and relevant recommendations about preventive services in primary care. For the USPSTF to recommend a service, the benefits of the service must outweigh the harms. The USPSTF focuses on maintenance of health and quality of life as the major benefits of clinical preventive services, and not simply the identification of disease. As a family physician, this is some of the staples of my profession—the prevention of disease. The USPSTF uses clinical evidence to generate treatment recommendations based on the available evidence. This is stratified into the following levels:

- Level I: Evidence obtained from at least one properly designed randomized controlled trial.

- Level II-1: Evidence obtained from well-designed controlled trials without randomization.

- Level II-2: Evidence obtained from well-designed cohort or case-control analytic studies, preferably from more than one center or research group.

- Level II-3: Evidence obtained from multiple time series with or without the intervention. Dramatic results in uncontrolled trials might also be regarded as this type of evidence.

- Level III: Opinions of respected authorities, based on clinical experience, descriptive studies, or reports of expert committees.

At first blush, the first thing that I notice is that despite all our best efforts, medical recommendations are still made based on the personal opinions of those with experience ("opinions of authorities" and "reports of committees"). I once sat on a committee, which provided guidance regarding policy making when I was in the navy. I guess stating that the "report of the brainstorming session" doesn't sound as professional. Regardless, it was the same thing. Modern medicine is not that modern, and recommendations are still based on personal experiences, as they have been for centuries. The take-home point is that medicine is not black and white. Sometimes the problem or treatment cannot be clearly defined. Anyone who feels otherwise can spend a week in my office. Sometimes the best answer I have for a problem is a Latin phrase that describes what I see. Sometimes treatment consists of "let's try this and see what happens." That's "modern medicine." The USPSTF, which is basis for many of Medicare's treatment or screening guidelines, understands that it is not an exact science quite yet. Unfortunately, not all entities do. This is evident with private insurances with the example of the asthma step therapy treatment plan, which, as you recall, is the recommendations of an "expert panel." As I have stated, many patients are held hostage, through step-therapy or prior authorization, to this algorithm even though it may not apply to them.

Unfortunately, I live with the downstream consequences of well-meaning clinical recommendations. Recommendations are just that, recommendations. They should not be taken as the one final and only treatment plan for a particular condition. One example is the recommendations that are associated with a diagnosis of diabetes. Some of the current recommendations for patients with diabetes are: they should receive an annual dilated eye exam from an ophthalmologist, they should be counseled on nutrition, they should have an annual foot exam to screen for nerve damage, they should have a specific blood test periodically to ensure good sugar control and to evaluate and treat other possible co-morbid conditions or complications, and certain medications should be considered to prevent or decrease risk of other medical problems, such as heart disease.[113] Again, sounds good in theory.

On any given day I receive three or four letters from insurance carriers entitled "clinical considerations." I call them practicing medicine. An example of a clinical consideration is something like the following phrase:

> Dear Provider, we have noticed that through billing data your patient has a diagnosis of [pick one, say diabetes]. According to our records, you have not performed a [pick your blood test] in the past twelve months. Please consider performing [said test or starting said medicine]. Please respond to this letter by completing the following questionnaire.

The "following questionnaire" subsequently consists of a six-page form in which I must justify my actions regarding the treatment of this patient. Often this requires a paragraph written to justify why I did or did not perform a particular action. There are many reasons why said action may or may not have been done. The most obvious is that it may not be clinically indicated in this patient. Patients have allergies, they are intolerant to certain medications, they may have other medical problems that conflict with the current recommendations, and so on. Now I am expected to write the equivalent of an essay as to why I did or did not do something based upon the results of data mining from the insurance company. Sometimes I get letters on patients that I have never seen. Insurance companies often will assign a "provider" to a patient, regardless of who the patient is actually seeing. It happens. I cannot evaluate someone whom I have not seen. Those wind up in the trash. But this gets even better, as soon as I talk about cars again.

I like to go back to the car analogy. In this case it's about deciding what kind of mechanic I want to be. Granted, I have been fortunate and do not have a lot of experience with mechanics, so my worldview may be skewed somewhat. This is in part because I had to fix my own cars when I was younger, and now I have a vehicle that requires little maintenance. Regardless, it seems there are roughly two types of garages and two types of mechanics. Either a mechanic is honest or he is not. I've dealt with both. Luckily, the vast majority has been honest with common sense, but I have also dealt with the other. Some will recommend maintenance that my vehicle does not need, or parts that do not need replacing. Some will over charge my auto insurance or me. I compare that to medical fraud. It's basically the same thing. Do I really need that cholesterol on a twenty-two-year-old with a previously normal one the year prior?

Then there's the garage. At a dealership, I am guaranteed an expensive diagnostic test before I can even explain why I brought the car there in the first place. Once there, they will be very thorough and find not only the problem but also numerous other potentially fixable problems, some of which may not be bothersome. If the mechanic is honest, then when I leave I will know that my car has been properly taken care of, whether it truly needed it or not. Then there's the local garage. The mechanic there will fix what is wrong. If there's something else glaringly obvious, then he will usually point it out to me and give me the option to get it fixed or not. He often can fix the problem that I came in with at a much lower cost than a dealership. The risk is that I may have something else break that we didn't address on the way home.

I try to keep both analogies in mind when I practice medicine. I certainly do not want to treat unnecessarily or overcharge, but I have to balance that with the need to be thorough. In medicine we only have one chance to screw up, and I have to get it right the first time. To accomplish this I have a frank and honest discussion with my patient. I try to remember my experiences with the mechanic when I am talking to the patient. If I were them, what would I want? What is the compromise, if any, between being overly cautious and expensive versus being too cavalier but less costly? I certainly do not recommend testing when it is unnecessary. Additionally, to what benefit is it to obtain diagnostic testing that is not clinically indicated ordered by individuals not qualified to interpret and manage the results? What do we gain when treatment options are limited?

So basically, I don't feel that I should be doing unnecessary things to people when it's not medically indicated, despite what that high school graduate working for that major insurance carrier thinks.

Today I can get away with that. Unfortunately, however, with the Pay for Performance model, I may be penalized if I use my best clinical judgment.

In the Pay for Performance (PFP) model, physicians, hospitals, medical groups, and other health care providers are rewarded financially for meeting certain performance measures for quality and efficiency and penalized for negative consequences of care or increased costs.[114] Most medical organizations agree, at least in part, that pay for performance can increase the quality of medical care, but there are reservations. The American Academy of Family Physicians, in a policy statement, states that the focus should be on a program which:

- Supports the physician/patient relationship

- Utilizes performance measures based on evidence-based clinical guidelines

- Involves practicing physicians in program design

- Uses reliable, accurate, and scientifically valid data

- Provides positive physician incentives

- Offers voluntary physician participation[115]

Unfortunately there are reservations. Overall, a Pay for Performance (PFP) should provide incentives to physician practices for:

- Adoption and utilization of health information technologies;

- Implementation of systems to improve the quality of patient care and patient safety;

- Adhering to evidence-based clinical guidelines;

- Improving performance and meeting performance targets;

- Improving patient access to appropriate and timely care; and

- Measuring and attempting to improve patient acceptance and satisfaction with their care.

However, this policy statement goes on to state that these programs should be consolidated across employers and health plans to make the payment meaningful and the program more manageable for physician practices. The administrative and financial burden of data mining and case management of basically entire towns can be cost prohibitive. The incentive programs should utilize new money funded by using a portion of the projected total system savings. There should be no reduction in existing fees for service paid to physicians as a result of implementing a PFP program. In other words, there should be no reduction in current fee payment with the incentive that, by meeting certain criteria, the fees will be "returned to normal." The financial rewards to physician practices must both recoup the additional administrative costs to participate in the program (data collection and measurement) and provide significant incentive. Medicine has become a "job" just like working at any other job. And after all, I'm pretty sure no one appreciates doing extra work for free.

The program cannot create incentives that place physicians at odds with their patients, e.g., incentives to fragment care or deselect certain patients. For example, if you refuse to exercise, lose weight, or take your medicine, then I as a physician should not be penalized for this. The likely response to this kind of penalty is that those "noncompliant" patients will not be able to find a physician who will be willing to see them. I cannot make people do something they do not want to do. Last I checked I still lived in America. Last I checked we are still free. People are free to choose what they wish to do or not do. If Susie wants to smoke two packs a day and develop lung cancer, she still has that right. It is my job to make sure she understands that her behavior is detrimental to her health, but I cannot physically stop her from smoking. My ability to support my family should not be dependent upon someone else's lifestyle choices.

Programs should minimize administrative, financial, and technological barriers to participation. In other words, if I have to hire an even larger team of case managers, computer operators, and billing specialists, that defeats the incentive of potentially higher revenue. The PFP entity should notify the patients affected, provide related self-care information, and reinforce patient responsibilities in achieving the desired health outcomes. If the insurance you participate in wants you in the program, they need to make the program and expectations very clear to you.

When evidence is lacking regarding the value of a particular diagnostic or therapeutic intervention, acknowledge that physicians' judgment, patient's preference, and the costs associated with various options may be the best measures of the appropriateness of a given intervention for PFP purposes. That seems pretty straightforward to me, but insurance company employees with checklists have already eroded that.

Patient cases should be removed from the performance measure when a physician can demonstrate that attempts have been made to provide patients support to follow recommended care, and they have subsequently not followed such recommendations, the recommendations are inappropriate for this patient due to other clinical or socioeconomic considerations, or the patient is unable to comply. Again, don't penalize the messenger.

Finally, programs should be designed to include practices of all sizes. Smaller practices should be able to participate as easily as large multispecialty groups. Of course, with the current trends in health care, there won't be too many small practices left anyway.

That leads me to the present.

# Present Health Care

In my average day, not only do I have to evaluate and treat thirty-plus people, I must report my findings to the appropriate third party entity. This can include the federal government, the state government, insurance carriers, lawyers who request medical information for various reasons, disability insurance carriers, and workman's compensation carriers. Thanks to HIPPA, this is done without your knowledge or consent. Let me give you some examples of what I currently have to do and report; then we shall discuss where we are going.

First of all, I need an electronic medical record system. Not only do I have to have a computer system with a huge startup cost and a few thousand dollars annually maintenance per physician, it must be able to transmit data and run reports appropriately. This is called Meaningful Use.

The requirements for Meaningful Use are summarized in an eighty-five-page document provided by the Center for Medicare and Medicaid Services (CMS).[116] Obviously, then, they are straightforward and easy to meet. All sarcasm aside, meeting the requirements for Meaningful Use in my office required hiring a full-time staff member to manage the program, thus increasing our overhead costs and patient overhead costs. Additionally, if I elect to decline participating, I am penalized. Medicare eligible professionals who do not meet the requirements for Meaningful Use by 2015 and in each subsequent year are subject to payment adjustments to their Medicare reimbursements that start at 1 percent per year, up to a maximum 5 percent annual adjustment.

Let me break this down some. Meaningful use can be summarized as requiring fifteen core objectives and ten menu objectives.

Core objectives are objectives that everyone who participates in the program must meet. Some of the core objectives have exclusions that could exempt a provider from having to meet them, but many of them do not. One must report on all fifteen core objectives and meet the thresholds established by those objectives. Providers need only to report on five out of the ten available menu objectives. In addition, eligible professionals have to report on clinical quality measures.

The following are the fifteen core objectives that every eligible professional must meet in order to receive an EHR incentive payment.

1.  Computerized provider order entry (CPOE)

2.  Drug-drug and drug-allergy checks

3.  Maintain an up-to-date problem list of current and active diagnoses

4.  E-Prescribing (eRx)

5.  Maintain active medication list

6.  Maintain active medication allergy list

7.  Record demographics

8.  Record and chart changes in vital signs

9.  Record smoking status for patients 13 years or older

10. Report ambulatory clinical quality measures to CMS/States

11. Implement clinical decision support

12. Provide patients with an electronic copy of their health information, upon request

13. Provide clinical summaries for patients for each office visit

14. Capability to exchange key clinical information

15. Protect electronic health information

Following the core objectives are the menu objectives. When selecting the five menu objectives, at least one must come from the Public Health list, which consists of the following:

1. Submit electronic data to immunization registries *or*

2. Submit electronic syndromic surveillance data to public health agencies.

After selecting a public health objective, four more menu objectives must be reported:

1. Drug formulary checks

2. Incorporate clinical lab-test results

3. Generate lists of patients by specific conditions

4. Send reminders to patients for preventive/follow-up care

5. Patient-specific education resources

6. Electronic access to health information for patients

7. Medication reconciliation

8. Summary of care record for transitions of care will have to report on:

    • three core clinical quality measures *and*

    • three clinical quality measures that you select from an additional list

Core measures include blood pressure measurement, preventive care and screening, and intervention for tobacco use, and adult weight screening and follow-up.

The clinical quality measures may be any three of the following:

1.  Diabetes: Hemoglobin A1c Poor Control

2.  Diabetes: Low Density Lipoprotein (LDL) Management and Control

3.  Diabetes: Blood Pressure Management

4.  Heart Failure (HF): Angiotensin-Converting Enzyme (ACE) Inhibitor or Angiotensin Receptor Blocker (ARB) Therapy for Left Ventricular Systolic Dysfunction (LVSD)

5.  Coronary Artery Disease (CAD): Beta-Blocker Therapy for CAD Patients with Prior Myocardial Infarction (MI)

6.  Pneumonia Vaccination Status for Older Adults

7.  Breast Cancer Screening

8.  Colorectal Cancer Screening

9.  Coronary Artery Disease (CAD): Oral Antiplatelet Therapy Prescribed for Patients with CAD

10. Heart Failure (HF): Beta-Blocker Therapy for Left Ventricular Systolic Dysfunction (LVSD)

11. Anti-Depressant Medication Management: (a) Effective Acute Phase Treatment, (b)Effective Continuation Phase Treatment

12. Primary Open Angle Glaucoma (POAG): Optic Nerve Evaluation

13. Diabetic Retinopathy: Documentation of Presence or Absence of Macular Edema and Level of Severity of Retinopathy

14. Diabetic Retinopathy: Communication with the Physician Managing Ongoing Diabetes Care

15. Asthma Pharmacologic Therapy

16. Asthma Assessment

17. Appropriate Testing for Children with Pharyngitis

18. Oncology Breast Cancer: Hormonal Therapy for Stage IC-IIIcEtrogen Receptor/Progesterone Receptor (ER/PR) Positive Breast Cancer

19. Oncology Colon Cancer: Chemotherapy for Stage III Colon Cancer Patients

20. Prostate Cancer: Avoidance of Overuse of Bone Scan for Staging Low Risk Prostate Cancer Patients

21. Smoking and Tobacco Use Cessation, Medical Assistance: a) Advising Smokers and Tobacco Users to Quit, b) Discussing Smoking and Tobacco Use Cessation Medications, c) Discussing Smoking and Tobacco Use Cessation Strategies

22. Diabetes: Eye Exam

23. Diabetes: Urine Screening

24. Diabetes: Foot Exam

25. Coronary Artery Disease (CAD): Drug Therapy for Lowering LDL-Cholesterol

26. Heart Failure (HF): Warfarin Therapy Patients with Atrial Fibrillation

27. Ischemic Vascular Disease (IVD): Blood Pressure Management

28. Ischemic Vascular Disease (IVD): Use of Aspirin or Another Antithrombotic

29. Initiation and Engagement of Alcohol and Other Drug Dependence Treatment:

30. Prenatal Care: Screening for Human Immunodeficiency Virus (HIV)

31. Prenatal Care: Anti-D Immune Globulin

32. Controlling High Blood Pressure

33. Cervical Cancer Screening

34. Chlamydia Screening for Women

35. Use of Appropriate Medications for Asthma

36. Low Back Pain: Use of Imaging Studies

37. Ischemic Vascular Disease (IVD): Complete Lipid Panel and LDL Control

38. Diabetes: Hemoglobin A1c Control (<8.0percent)

But wait; there is more than one stage to Meaningful Use. The guidelines for stage two, released in August of 2012, expand the guidelines of electronic medical record use. In a handy 672-page document, CMS defines the requirements for Meaningful Use stage two.[117] This stage in part increases the reporting requirements for eligible providers. Justification for this is that certified technology used in a meaningful way is one piece of a broader health information technology infrastructure needed to reform the health care system and improve health care quality, efficiency, and patient safety.

But wait...

Physician Quality Reporting System formerly known as the Physician Quality Reporting Initiative is a reporting program that uses a combination of incentive payments and payment adjustments to promote reporting of quality information by eligible professionals.[118] The program provides an incentive payment to practices with eligible professionals (identified on claims by their individual National Provider Identifier [NPI] and Tax Identification Number [TIN]) who satisfactorily report data on quality measures for covered Physician Fee Schedule (PFS) services furnished to Medicare Part B Fee-for-Service (FFS) beneficiaries (including Railroad Retirement Board and Medicare Secondary Payer). Beginning in 2015, the program also applies a payment adjustment to eligible professionals who do not satisfactorily report data on quality measures for covered professional services. Reporting quality measures data via one of the reporting mechanisms above for services furnished during a 2012 reporting period will qualify to earn a Physician Quality Reporting incentive payment equal to 0.5 percent of their total estimated Medicare Part B Physician Fee Schedule (PFS) allowed charges for covered professional services furnished during that same reporting period.

There is no current requirement to participate in the PQRI. However, CMS finalized in its 2012 Medicare Physician Fee Schedule that 2015 program penalties will be based on 2013 performance. Therefore, those physicians who elect not to participate or are found unsuccessful during the 2013 program year will receive a 1.5 percent payment penalty, and 2 percent thereafter. The American Medical Association (AMA) is strongly advocating for removal of PQRI penalties, and specifically the linking of 2015 program penalties with 2013 performance.[119] The results of this remain to be seen.

The measures in 2012 Physician Quality Reporting address various aspects of care, such as prevention, chronic- and acute-care management, procedure-related care, resource utilization, and care coordination.

These measures consist of two major components: a denominator that describes the eligible cases for a measure (the eligible patient population associated with a measure's numerator), and a numerator that describes the clinical action required by the measure for reporting and performance.

Each component is defined by specific codes described in each measure specification along with reporting instructions and use of modifiers. There are 316 reportable quality measures to choose from. For now, an individual physician must report three or more measures to receive the incentive payment (or to not be penalized). I suspect this number will creep up slowly as the system becomes more refined until most every disease state will have to be reported in one form or the other. Recall, the HIPPA act loosened the restraints on the release of health care information such that this information now flows freely out of my computer onto the government databases where it is analyzed, my performance picked apart based upon a "standardized" treatment protocol, and both you and I receive a "grade." For me, the consequences relate to the amount of payment I receive or how much I am penalized from an insurance company. For you, that potentially translates to what you will wind up paying in insurance premiums.

Electronic Prescribing (eRx) Incentive Program. The Electronic Prescribing (eRx) Incentive Program is a reporting program that uses a combination of incentive payments and payment adjustments to encourage electronic prescribing by eligible professionals.[120] The program provides an incentive payment to practices with eligible professionals (identified on claims by their individual National Provider Identifier [NPI] and Tax Identification Number [TIN]) who successfully e-prescribe for covered Physician Fee Schedule (PFS) services furnished to Medicare Part B Fee-for-Service (FFS) beneficiaries (including Railroad Retirement Board and Medicare Secondary Payer). Beginning in 2012, the program also applies a payment adjustment to those eligible professionals who are not successful electronic prescribers on their Medicare Part B services. Translation: those who do not meet the requirements are penalized.

In order to report this measure, a qualified electronic prescribing (eRx) system must have been adopted. To "adopt" an eRx system, I must pay a startup cost of somewhere around five thousand dollars in addition to monthly maintenance in the hundreds of dollars. CMS then determines whether the eligible professional has adopted a "qualified" eRx system and the extent of its use. A "qualified" eRx system is one that is capable of all of the following functionalities:

a.  Generate a complete active medication list incorporating electronic data received from applicable pharmacies and pharmacy benefit managers (PBMs) if available.

b.  Select medications, print prescriptions, electronically transmit prescriptions, and conduct alerts. This functionality *must* be enabled.

c.  Provide information related to lower cost or therapeutically appropriate alternatives (if any).

d.  Provide information on formulary or tiered formulary medications, patient eligibility, and authorization requirements received electronically from the patient's drug plan (if available).

For successful reporting under the 2012 eRx Incentive Program, a single quality-data code (eRx G-code) should be reported, according to the following coding and reporting principles:

a.  Report the following eRx numerator G-code, when applicable: G8553- At least one prescription created during the encounter was generated and transmitted electronically using a qualified eRx system (faxes do not count).

b.  The eRx G-code, which supplies the numerator, must be reported: o on the claim(s) with the denominator billing code(s) that represent the eligible encounter for the 2012 eRx incentive payment; or on the claim(s) with any billing code(s) that represent the encounter to avoid the 2013 eRx payment adjustment:

    •  for the same beneficiary

    •  for the same date of service (DOS)

- by the same eligible professional (individual NPI) who performed the covered service as the payment codes, usually CPT Category I or HCPCS codes, which supply the denominator.

c. For purposes of reporting the eRx G-code to avoid the 2013 eRx payment adjustment, the eRx G-code can be reported on the claim(s) during the reporting period, regardless of whether the code for such service appears in the denominator.

- The eRx G-code must be submitted with a line-item charge of zero dollars ($0.00) at the time the associated covered service is performed:

- The submitted charge field cannot be blank.

- The line-item charge should be $0.00.

- If a system does not allow a $0.00 line-item charge, a nominal amount, such as $0.01, can be substituted —the beneficiary is not liable for this nominal amount.

- Whether a $0.00 charge or a nominal amount is submitted to the Carrier/Medicare Administrative Contractor (MAC), the eRx G-code line is denied and tracked.

That brings me to the reporting code. A reporting code is a procedure code that is sent, via the billing process for tracking purposes. For a typical Medicare patient, I must process on any given day upward of eight procedure codes for routine reporting. This includes such information as whether or not you are obese, what your blood pressure is, if you received a prescription, whether or not you have had a bone density test looking for osteoporosis and if not why, whether you smoke or not, and what your sugar and cholesterol is. That is mandatory. If I do not do this, I am potentially financially penalized.

I hope the previous guidelines have not confused you. I must report all these all the time at the time of your office appointment, even if you come in for an annoying rash and ask me out at the same time. Failure to do so will result in penalties. Oh, and I have to also actually take care of the reason why you are on my exam table (the rash, of course).

Medicare in 2012 also decided that preventive care is important. When CMS finds something important, that roughly translates as it becomes a reimbursable/payable item—herding cats after all. When a Medicare beneficiary presents to my office for preventive care, I have one of three choices. The patient is either new to the Medicare system, the patient is not new to the Medicare system but has not undergone a Medicare preventive exam, or the patient is returning for a follow-up preventive exam. So far it doesn't seem too difficult. Let's delve into the reporting requirements. In addition to all of the above requirements, I must report the following:

The patient new to Medicare, also called the "welcome to Medicare" physical, requires the following elements: the initial EKG and the associated reporting code; the Medicare physical code; a vision screen and any other age-appropriate screening tests, which can include a lipid panel, metabolic panel, prostate screening (which is controversial), appropriate immunizations, and screening for colon cancer and aortic aneurysm for those who meet the requirements. I must also document counseling on end-of-life planning, do a depression screen, review modifiable risk factors for disease detection (whatever that means), and discuss safety/education. Those are all "covered" services. The ironic part is that if one would get the welcome to Medicare physical, it would go almost 100 percent toward the annual deductible, thus costing Medicare nothing.

In addition to the welcome to Medicare physical, I can also perform the initial and (the following years) the subsequent annual examination. In these examinations, I must screen for: diabetes, aortic aneurysm when appropriate, alcoholism, colon cancer, depression, HIV, high blood pressure, high cholesterol, need for aspirin therapy, obesity, syphilis (I've never seen a case of syphilis), other sexually transmitted diseases, calculate risk of death, determine end-of-life planning, screen for cervical cancer, genetic risk for breast cancer, breast cancer itself, osteoporosis, and dementia. The reporting documentation guidelines are specific and require a diagnosis code as well as a procedure code.

Typically I screen these for appropriateness when the patient normally comes in for an annual examination. However, given the reporting requirements, I must now employ an additional staff member to assist in completing the reporting requirements, again increasing patient overhead and increasing overall health care costs.

The future requires even more reporting and more third party intervention. The future requires that my office be certified, and the Patient Centered Medical Home (PCMH) is the future of primary care. The PCMH is a team-based health care delivery model led by a physician that provides comprehensive and continuous medical care to patients with the goal of obtaining maximized health outcomes.[121] The rationale is that this model of health care delivery may allow better access to health care, increase satisfaction with care, and improve health. Care coordination is an essential component of the PCMH. Unfortunately, care coordination requires additional resources such as health information technology and appropriately trained staff to provide coordinated care through team-based models.

It is becoming more recognized that primary care is a foundation of the health care system. The PCMH program gives practices information about organizing care around patients, working in teams, and coordinating and tracking care over time. Primary care clinicians are often the first point of contact for an individual; thus, patient access to care is an important issue in this model. Primary care physicians must have a broad knowledge of many health care conditions and often follow their patients over years; thus, the quality of the clinician/patient relationship and the physicians' ability to track care over time is important. Primary care clinicians also sometimes need to refer patients to specialists. Communication among the referring and referred provider is important and often challenging and is also emphasized in the PCMH model.

In this methodology, systems are designed to facilitate partnerships between individual patients, their personal physicians, and when appropriate the patient's family. Using registries, information technology, health information exchange, and other means to assure that patients get the "indicated care" when and where they need and want it in an appropriate manner coordinates care.[122]

That translates as reporting your medical information, possibly to third party entities, for management. Currently in my office, I have an employee whose job description includes running reports from the electronic medical record database. These reports may include such things as patients who are past due on mammograms, cholesterol checks, or whether someone has been appropriately counseled on some disease state or the other. Once the report is generated, it is given to another employee who then makes calls and coordinates care. Independent of the PCMH model, I already routinely receive third party reports on which "clinical care consideration" I am delinquent on this week. Third party entities include, of course, insurance companies, the government, and possibly in the future other as-of-yet uncreated private entities whose sole responsibility is to gather data and subsequently tell me what I should do with my patients. Last I checked in my home state of Indiana, that is practicing medicine (of course, without any responsibility or liability), but I'm just a doctor, not a lawyer, so maybe I'm incorrect in this assumption.

The PCMH is a process. To become a certified "medical home," an office must comply with the standards designed by, and pay money to, a certifying body. My office follows the guidelines of my specialty academy and we are using NCQA (National

Committee for Quality Assurance) standards. In addition to pay-ing our three thousand dollar application fee, I must demonstrate that the practice is compliant with the certification standards.[123] My reporting requirements are not only numerous and onerous, but are in addition to the mandatory reporting requirements of PQRS, eRx, Meaningful Use, and Medicare preventative exami-nation reporting.

The upside to this is that if practices achieve NCQA's PCMH Recognition, they can take advantage of financial incentives that health plans, employers, federal- and state-sponsored pilot pro-grams offer. Furthermore, they may qualify for additional bonuses or payments.

In order to attain PCMH Recognition, specific elements must be met. Included in the standards are ten must-pass elements:[124]

- Access and communication processes: The practice has written processes for scheduling appointments and com-municating with patients.

- Access and communication results: The practice has data showing that it meets the standards in element 1A for scheduling and communicating with patients.

- Organizing clinical data: The practice uses electronic or paper-based charting tools to organize and document clinical information.

- Identifying important conditions: The practice uses an electronic or paper-based system to identify the follow-ing in the practice's patient population: most frequently seen diagnoses, most important risk factors, three clini-cally important conditions.

- Guidelines for important conditions: The practice must implement evidence-based guidelines for the three iden-tified clinically important conditions.

- Self-management support: The practice works to facilitate self-management of care for patients with one of the three clinically important conditions.

- Test tracking and follow-up: The practice works to improve effectiveness of care by managing the timely receipt of information on all tests and results.

- Referral tracking: The practice seeks to improve effectiveness, timeliness, and coordination of care by following through on critical consultations with other practitioners.

- Measures of performance: The practice measures or receives performance data by physician or across the practice regarding: clinical process, clinical outcomes, service data, patient safety.

- Reporting to physicians: The practice reports on its performance on the factors in referral tracking.

For each element there are numerous sub standards (called factors) that must be met. There are a total of 162 possible factors, but not all must be met to be certified as a medical home. Imagine the administrative burden of generating these reports. Now imagine that I am dealing with this, above and beyond trying to actually do my job and figure out what is wrong with you and how I am going to fix it. Now imagine that the guy two appointments before you was a douche.

Two days ago in the office a glorious thing happened. Our office server crashed. It was a total meltdown. They said it will take a week to rebuild. At first the staff and patients were dismayed and confused. Many of our staff had never worked without the computer system.

The veteran office staff shrugged, pulled out a piece of paper, and the following tragedy happened: nothing.

Patients were still seen. They were actually seen in a more timely fashion, because there was not the obligatory demographic data input. No insurance cards were verified in real time, no photos were taken. No kiosk data input was entered. Front office information was written down on the billing requisition and passed to the assistants. Vitals and ancillary tests such as EKGs and lung function tests were performed the old-fashioned way with manual equipment and printed to paper. Medical assistants obtained the history and prepared the patient. And I had the luxury of doing what I went into medicine to do. Talk to people, listen to them, and help them. I was not preoccupied with reporting the status of their disease state to the authorities or fight others trying to play doctor. In the exam room it was only my patient and me. On those days I actually practiced medicine. It lasted two weeks. Then I was tasked with the creation of all the reporting data that was not incorporated into the system during that time.

So what's next? The next step is to incorporate the PCMH concept into the medical organization as a whole. This gives rise to the Accountable Care Organization (ACO). An ACO is a health care organization characterized by a payment and care delivery model that seeks to tie provider reimbursements to quality metrics and reductions in the total cost of care for an assigned population of patients.[125] The ACO is accountable to the patients and the third-party payer for the quality, appropriateness, and efficiency of the health care provided. Of course, how does one verify accountability? By running reporting data, that's how. Good thing I already run a dozen or so reports daily. ACOs will be the future of health care.

One working example of an ACO is the Veteran's Administration System. This hallowed yet arguably underfunded institution (of which I am not eligible to receive care despite sixteen years of military service) institutes the ACO's team model of health care delivery. As stated by *The Washington Monthly*, in a study published in the New England Journal of Medicine in 2003, VA health facilities, when compared to other fee-for-service Medicare institutions, provided significantly better care when measured on eleven quality indicators. Additionally, it stated that the Annals of Internal Medicine also published a study that compared veterans' health facilities with commercial managed-care systems in their treatment of diabetes patients. In seven out of seven measures of quality, the VA provided better care.[126] One may only need to look as far as the neighborhood VA facility to see the future.

# What a Pain: Chronic Pain and Primary Care

I want to touch briefly on the topic of chronic pain and pain medication. The misuse, abuse, and trafficking of prescription medication, especially narcotic painkillers, is a huge problem. Tens of thousands of Americans die each year currently from prescription drug abuse. According to the Center for Disease Control, prescription drugs are responsible for more overdose deaths than "street drugs" such as cocaine, heroin, and amphetamines, while the number of emergency room visits attributable to pharmaceuticals alone was up 97 percent between 2004 and 2008.[127]

In June of 2010 Slipknot bassist Paul Gray died by accidental overdose of prescription painkillers. His physician, Dr Daniel Baldi, was charged with involuntary manslaughter and faces up to sixteen years in prison if convicted. Slipknot released a press release that stated, in part, "As the loss of our brother Paul Gray is still very fresh for us in the Slipknot family, this new development has us all in a state of anger and sadness…We plan to cooperate as much as we possibly can to ensure this tragedy is never repeated and to make sure this man pays for what he has done."[128]

From a physician's standpoint, pain management is a very difficult problem legally, ethically, and medically.

First of all, let me start with the fact that people lie. It is a known fact. How much do you smoke? How much do you exercise? How much do you drink? Now, how much do you really drink? It's probably a lot more than you told me, I guarantee. No worries, because as a physician it is my job to pick up on nonverbal cues, and I'm fairly good at knowing when someone is trying to pull the wool over my eyes. If I'm suspicious of your answer, I usually just mentally adjust the number you told me, and I move on. It's a game, and we all know how it's played.

Pain is a different animal, and "drug seekers" are entirely different altogether. I have had patients tell me whatever they think I want to hear to get a prescription. I won't give an example here, since to some extent there is a pattern to this, and I can over time ferret out the seekers from legitimate pain sufferers. I don't want to give away all my trade secrets. Some of people will look me right in the eye and completely lie to me with a smile on their face.

In addition to that, sociopathic behavior and sometimes-uncontrolled mental illness is very difficult to address in a ten-minute appointment slot. More than once irate patients have knocked over equipment or left my office yelling when I refused to prescribe narcotics. I personally do not have a "no weapons" policy in the office. If a seeker decides to start shooting, at least I can hope for return fire from law enforcement and concerned citizens. Out of patient necessity, I do see a few limited patients for chronic pain management. Out of personal necessity, I also have a concealed weapons permit. And yes, I do know how to shoot.

Pain is subjective. Clearly if you have just mauled off a good chunk of your leg with a chainsaw, that hurts. Unfortunately, not all pain can be easily identified. How bad does a herniated disk hurt? I don't know. I don't have one. We often use the pain scale.[129] On a scale of one to ten, how bad does it hurt? Invariably the answer is eleven. Okay, that's useless. So here's my conundrum: A patient wanders into my office. He has an MRI showing a bad disk in his back. It's not so bad that he needs surgery, but it's not so mild that I disbelieve what he is telling me. What do I do with this patient who is writhing in pain in my office? What about Grandma has severe arthritis and is not a surgical candidate? She cannot take anti-inflammatories or acetaminophen. Her grand-child is more than helpful in preparing her pills for the week, and some months she mysteriously comes up short. Do I deny her pain medication? There are many other scenarios that I could demonstrate, but the point is, not everything is black and white.

I have a moral obligation to treat my patients to the best of my ability and in their best interest. In a perfect world I could refer any in question to a surgical specialist who could provide definitive treatment or refer to a pain management specialist. Unfortunately, under the watchful eye of the DEA and other law enforcement agencies, pain management physicians are extremely difficult to find, and it's even harder to get a patient in to be seen. Also, after a patient has failed therapy, surgeries, and pain blocks by specialists, they are returned to my care. That brings me back to square one.

Laws differ from state to state in regards to controlled sub-stances, which are medications, that are generally considered as having the potential for abuse or addiction. In my state, we have a state registry which tracks all controlled substance prescriptions filled. I also have access to the controlled substance registries of two neighboring states. That helps considerably. Within a few minutes I can see if someone has filled multiple prescriptions by different physicians, which is called "doctor shopping." It also helps identify providers who prescribe excessive amounts of nar-cotics. The licensing board of my state then can, if necessary, take appropriate actions if there is an unscrupulous provider.

An old-fashioned bottle of acetaminophen bought at the con-venient store that many of us have in our medicine cabinet has enough toxic potential to kill someone numerous times over.[130] The medication is safe and effective when taken as directed, but when misused it can lead to a slow, painful death via liver failure. Many pain medications contain acetaminophen and when prescribed appropriately, are safe and effective. When they are combined with other forms of acetaminophen, the combination can be deadly.

In 2005, twenty-eight billion doses of acetaminophen containing products were purchased in the United States, of which eight billion were acetaminophen alone. From 1998 to 2003, acetaminophen was the leading cause of acute liver failure in the United States, and it is estimated that there are about 1,600 cases of liver failure, of which the most common cause was acetaminophen-related, each year. In addition to death, in the decade of the 1900s, there were an estimated 56,000 emergency room visits, 26,000 hospitalizations, and 458 deaths related to acetaminophen-associated overdoses.

The question becomes, then, what is the definition of excessive amounts of narcotics? Who makes that determination? Me, or is it the state, the DEA, the prosecuting attorney, the judge, or an angry mob?

A disturbing trend that I see developing, like everything else in medicine, is third party involvement interfering in the physician-patient relationship. In 2012, Kentucky proposed House Bill 481. This bill, sponsored by John Tilley, D-Hopkinsville, proposed beefing up the attorney general's power to police overprescribing of narcotics by health care providers.[131] All health care practitioners would have to use the Kentucky All Schedule Prescription Electronic Reporting, or KASPER, before prescribing Schedule II or III narcotics. Medications are rated, or scheduled, based upon the abuse and addiction potential. A schedule II is worse than a schedule III or IV. The attorney general's office, not the Cabinet for Health and Family Services, which currently monitors this program, would oversee the KASPER program. The reasoning stated is that the move is needed to make the database a more effective law enforcement tool. Note that the emphasis on this is as a law enforcement tool rather than as a tool to help practitioners and the state licensing agency curb the over pre-scribing by physicians and doctor shopping by seekers.

In addition to making the practice of medicine a criminal offense, the attorney general would be able to charge a fee to health care providers to maintain and operate the monitoring sys-tem. Any law enforcement officer could access the system's records after certifying that he or she is part of a legitimate investigation, which I suspect falls under the auspices of the HIPPA law, allow-ing any "interested party" free and total access to medical records.

We are now back to the exam room and the patient writhing on my exam table. I could treat you with pain medication, but in doing so I risk going to jail and losing my medical license. I could not treat you. Morally that is not the right answer. Plus it's also risky from a liability standpoint.

In 2001, a California jury found an internist, Wing Chin, MD, liable for under-treating pain.[132] The jurors found him guilty of elder abuse and recklessness and awarded the now-deceased man's family 1.5 million dollars. The guilty verdict came even though he prescribed Demerol (a narcotic) to eighty-five-year-old William Bergman to ease the back pain he complained of when he arrived at the Eden Medical Center in Castro Valley, California, in 1998. Dr. Chin sent Bergman home with Vicodin and a skin patch containing another narcotic. Dr. Chin used those painkillers after a dose of morphine temporarily stopped Bergman's breath-ing. Bergman's children said the painkillers their father received weren't strong enough, because he was given a fraction of the normal dosage. On a one to ten scale with ten being the worst, he ranked his pain between seven and ten during his six-day hospi-tal stay. Consequently, they said, he suffered unnecessarily during his final days battling cancer. The family said it sued so that doc-tors would be more diligent about treating patients' pain.

So now let's take that scenario and move to the exam room. Under-treat and I'm potentially negligent. Over-treat and I'm criminally liable and going to jail. Not treat at all and I'm not following my oath as a physician.

# Voodoo 101 and You

No One Gets In To See The Wizard! Not no one, not no
how!

—Wizard of Oz 1939

In my office, the central reception area is an open circle. In this
area patients are checked in, checked out, payments are collected,
and the phones answered. Our staff is trained to perform all these
tasks, so depending on the ebb and flow of patients in the waiting
room, they can reduce any potential bottleneck in patient flow.
Regardless, I pass by this hub, as we call it, on my way to the
kitchenette where I drink entirely too much coffee throughout
the day. Invariably one of staff members is on the phone scheduling an appointment. The question they ask is, "Which doctor
would you like to see?" I answer them as I walk by, "I prefer the
term Shaman, not witch-doctor." Regardless, let's roll the bones.

The Hippocratic Oath charges me to teach future generations. I could teach rotating medical students and residents how
to evaluate and treat any number of disease states. However, I like
to teach them voodoo. In my office we roll the proverbial bones
and peer into hearts and minds of humanity to affect positive
change. That's a responsibility that shouldn't be taken lightly, and
I try to teach them what can't be found in a textbook.

As with anything, we humans have expectations. Some of these are reasonable, and some, especially in medicine, less so. Expectations can turn the same experience into a good one or a bad experience. Is a thirty-minute wait time a good thing or a bad thing? That depends on whether you expected to wait an hour or expected to walk right back to the exam room.

By understanding patient expectations, a physician can provide better care.[133] Patient satisfaction is, of course, one of the goals of medicine. As a product line of the service industry, physicians must increasingly understand and be attentive to the needs of our clients, in these case patients. The old timers in my office bristle at the notion that the role of a physician has deteriorated from the hallowed and noble profession of Hippocrates to a product line of the same caliber as my neighborhood barber or they guy who drives around my neighborhood selling frozen food out of his truck, but whatever. It's a job.

But what kind of expectations do we have as patients? Personally, when I go to the doctor, I enjoy that metallic smell from those iodine-based cleaners. I don't have any of that smelly sanitizer stuff in my office, and my exam rooms usually just smell like whichever air freshener we are using that day. Some expectations are as simple as my appearance. In one study the data suggest that age and style of dress are important considerations in a patient's ability to trust a physician. The majority of patients stated a preference for their doctors to be between thirty and fifty years old, and it preferred a male physician to dress in the traditional "professional" manner with a white coat, tie, shirt, and dress pants. In another study, individuals judge the quality and qualifications of psychotherapists by the way their offices look.

One of the questions that I always ask a resident rotating with me is simply, "What do they want?" What is this particular patient's expectation coming into this visit? The answer is deceptive, both simple and quite complex simultaneously. The answer can be as simple as a work note, or it can be as complicated as wanting me to wave a magic wand or sprinkle fairy dust and make their entire medical and social problems disappear. Often, though, it's much more basic: E&E: Empathy and Explanation.[134]

Patients must feel that their physician has listened to them. [135] That's difficult to teach a resident. Either the person has the inherent social skills to navigate the primary care arena, or they have their own daytime television show or peddle diet plans. Real doctors don't have time for that nonsense. Our obligation to our patients consumes our lives. Medicine is a jealous mistress. We barely have time to sleep.

Additionally, we all want an explanation. Without an explanation, what I do is "voodoo" magic just as electromagnetism seems magical until one understands how and why it works. The explanation must be understandable as well. Reiterating the Latin phrase for whatever the condition is does not explain anything. Why is this here? What caused it? What will make it go away? What are the consequences of having something like this? Why do I need to take an aspirin? Why should I spend the equivalent of a used car on a diagnostic test that will likely be normal? Those are the kinds of questions that must be answered. One of my patient teaching tools, for example, is drawing a picture of what I am trying to explain.

With the adoption of the PCMH, Meaningful Use, and the other programs that encompass medicine, there is increased emphasis on increasing access to the physician. I can now be formally contacted electronically via an Internet patient portal into my medical record system, I can be sent faxes, be called during working hours, and be called after hours. The expectation is becoming more and more that patients will have unlimited and immediate access to me at all hours of the day and night. That would be fine if I didn't do any of the following: see other patients in the office, sleep, eat, shower, watch my kids' school plays or sporting events, read a book, go grocery shopping, or basically do anything that one might consider normal living outside of work.

A trip to the grocery store will result in at least one or two clinical questions. More than once I was obligated to practice medicine while shopping and have called in prescriptions from the bread aisle. It is not uncommon for patient requests, such as making or cancelling appointments, at odd times when I am not in a position to oblige. More than once I have had to explain that I am currently at my son's soccer practice and I am sure that if they would call back during normal office hours we can address the issue appropriately.

Daily I receive phone calls from patients who just want to "ask me a few questions." As much as I would like to oblige them, I cannot. My primary assistant is a great resource in this matter, and if there is a problem that she cannot handle, then an appointment is probably in order. I cannot drop everything to answer a phone call simply because my time during office hours is designed to see other patients who have an office visit. As a proud product line in the service industry, what is it that I actually sell? A carpenter sells his ability to build, and a barber his ability to cut hair. Simply, I sell my time and my expertise. Phone calls, messages, and effective communication in general are vital components to medicine. I want to know if a medicine is causing problems or if symptoms change. I want to know that you picked up your medicine or had the surgery. However, there is a line. With increasing deductibles and the soaring cost of health care, more and more calls are patients wanting me to "call something in" without a proper evaluation. By merely describing their symptoms over the phone, I am expected to appropriately evaluate, diagnose, and treat the condition. Oh, and for free. The improper use of a telephone conversation to attempt to avoid the office visit is not only a medically dangerous thing to do; it also is akin to shoplifting. It is obtaining goods (prescriptions) or services (medical advice) without paying for it.

Lawyers as a profession understand this. I found out through firsthand experience that any interaction with Counsel is a billable service. This includes phone calls, e-mails, and personal visits, down to the postage spent to send a letter. I cannot do this nor do I wish to, because it increases barriers to effective communication. However, expectations must align more with reality for the system to work properly. Unrealistic expectations result in dissatisfied patients, but regardless, no one sees the wizard without an appointment.

# Health Department and Public Health: Dwindling Resources and Increased Demands

As health officer for my county, I am in charge of the health department. The health department's primary responsibilities include residential sewage disposal, retail food inspections, vital records, public health nursing, housing, vector control, emergency preparedness, and nuisance issues.[136] The authority to address these public health and safety issues frequently exceeds that of the State Department of Health. Unfortunately, the execution of this responsibility becomes more difficult as budgets are tightened and duties increase with the growing local population.

One responsibility in particular is that of our maternal child clinic. This is a clinic that provides family-related health services and little or no cost to a family based on their income. Services include annual exams, prenatal exams, birth control methods, screenings, and education.

This project is supported in part by Title V Maternal and Child Health Block Grant funds administered through the Indiana State Department of Health.[137] Enacted in 1935 as a part of the Social Security Act, the Title V Maternal and Child Health Program is the nation's oldest federal-state partnership. For over seventy-five years, the Federal Title V Maternal and Child Health program has provided a foundation for ensuring the health of the nation's mothers, women, children and youth, including children and youth with special health care needs, and their families. States and jurisdictions must match every four dollars of Federal Title V money that they receive by at least three dollars of state and/or local money. This "match" results in more than six billion dollars being available annually for maternal and child health programs at the state and local levels. At least 30 percent of Federal Title V funds are earmarked for preventive and primary care services for children, and at least 30 percent are earmarked for services for children with special health care needs.

With the future of the entire Social Security program in question, we are scrambling to make this clinic in my county as self-sufficient as possible so that we can continue to provide these much-needed services to our residents. Additionally, without a match from the state, the federal money may not be available. Although the population in Indiana has grown by almost a half million over the past decade, expenditure for health care has remained flat. Unfortunately, the start-up burden of electronic medical records, electronic prescribing requirements, electronic billing, and the subsequent ongoing monthly maintenance and interface fees of these services are prohibitively expensive. All we can do at this point is try to prepare as best we can and hope the funding does not dry up.

# Defensive Medicine

I was shopping the other day when I was approached by a patient of mine in the parking lot. Now, this isn't an unusual occurrence, but what followed was.

Patient: "Hey, Doc!"

Me: "Hey, wassup?"

Patient: "I know you can't talk about other patients, but you can listen, right?"

Me, thinking: *This is gonna be good.*

Me, saying: "Sure."

Patient: "Well, you know that So-and-so is your patient, right? I don't like talking about other people, but I feel that I need to warn you. They are my next-door neighbors, and they are sue-happy. Just wanted to warn you."

Me: "Oh, thanks."

A week later I received a subpoena for records in regards to a medical malpractice lawsuit aimed at a surgeon to whom I had referred the patient.

Defensive medicine is, in a nutshell, also called "Cover Your Ass" (CYA) medicine. Every patient encounter, whether it be an office visit, hospital rounds, or phone call, are all potential malpractice cases. Every office note that is now written is with the expectation that the note will be subpoenaed for a lawsuit of one kind or the other. I must prove or disprove every diagnosis or potentially life-threatening diagnosis using objective evidence of some sort, whether it is a lab test, diagnostic study, or second opinion, regardless of whether I needed the test to make the diagnosis. After all, I have an 87 percent chance of getting sued.

As an example, one of the leading reasons for a malpractice suit in primary care is a missed colon cancer. So I have a patient, we will call her Miranda, who presents to the office with an anemia. She is a chubby redhead with very heavy periods. Her blood work suggests an iron deficiency anemia based on what is called the red blood cell indices. Her red cells are smaller than average due to an iron deficiency, which I would expect in a red head with heavy periods.

Unfortunately, colon cancer can cause slow bleeding and subsequently an anemia that looks like her anemia. The question becomes, then, does everyone with an anemia, regardless of probable cause, warrant a colonoscopy? The short answer in this case is yes, of course. I have personally not ever detected a colon cancer based upon an isolated anemia found or routine blood work, but I guarantee if you present with a new anemia, you are getting your colon looked at.

Another example that I see weekly is pneumonia. If a patient presents with what appears to be classic community acquired pneumonia, is a chest X-ray (CXR) warranted? If I did a chest X-ray and it is normal, will it change the management of the patient? The answer is no. Although antibiotics are not "officially" warranted in a patient with bronchitis, whose crystal ball is working? Mine is in the shop. I don't know if this will blossom into pneumonia after a few days and some hydration or if this will remain bronchitis. Regardless, the question is, do I do a CXR to rule in a pneumonia or not? If I did a CXR and it showed pneumonia, I am now obligated to repeat another in about six weeks to ensure clearing of the infiltrate while exposing the patient to more radiation. If I do not repeat the study and the patient winds up at some point in the future having a lung cancer, which happens frequently enough, did I fail to diagnose? What happens when the patient had pneumonia on CXR but failed to show up for his repeat X-ray? What if don't do an X-ray at all? What if the patient doesn't have insurance? Is a diagnostic test that potentially could cost a hundred dollars or so needed even though it won't change the management of the patient? Those questions must be answered in the exam room.

Having trained in the navy, I was taught to use my eyes, ears, and hands to diagnose and treat patients. With some exceptions, most diagnostic tests that I run routinely are not to help me evaluate and treat the patient. They are used as stepping stones to management, to "prove" the clinical impression so that I can take the next step in treatment or to disprove a diagnosis for liability purposes. Unfortunately, this obligation to prove or disprove a diagnosis despite my professional clinical impression can sometimes be costly and, of course, is not without inherent risk. Primum non nocere does not apply when I am trying to cover my ass.

With regards to treatment, unfortunately, this next step often involves the participation of a specialist such as a surgeon or a treatment that I have to get authorized through the insurance company. Neither will just take my word for it. A neurosurgeon won't even schedule an appointment without an MRI, and I can't get an MRI unless the patient has had an X-ray first and the subsequent unnecessary radiation. I can't prescribe certain respiratory medicines unless I can produce a test showing what I already figured was wrong in the first place. I must demonstrate either objective proof of the diagnosis or have shown the algorithmic step-wise process that will lead me to the treatment plan that I am looking for.

The other reason for potentially unnecessary testing again is to disprove a diagnosis. Examples include coronary artery disease in a patient who presents with atypical symptoms, which are attributable to anxiety, or a CT scan to rule out appendicitis or other intra-abdominal process in a patient with probable irritable bowel disease. I receive numerous records requests from law firms every single day. I do not have the right to remain silent. HIPPA says that I must cough up my medical records, and I am acutely aware that everything I say and do, or don't do for that matter, can and will be used against me in a court of law.

# How's Your Day?

In my experience, there is a misconception that if I am not available to take a phone call or drop whatever I am doing to see Grandma in the nursing home, I am on my yacht or on the golf course. I don't play golf. That takes four hours. I don't have four hours.

Let me share with you a typical week for me. In my practice, there are seven of us who take call. That works out to call for our clinic patients about once a week during the weekday and about every fifth weekend depending if someone is out of town or whatnot. Call for the office consists of returning calls from patients who have questions or concerns after hours. Legitimate calls include the ubiquitous baby with a fever, random bleeding and/or pain, etc. Not so legitimate calls at 3:00 a.m. include the seeker with the narcotic pain medication request, calling to cancel or schedule an appointment, calling to get routine results, or reporting a power outage as our office number differs from the electric company by only one digit. I also take call for the hospital. This averages about the same amount of call. Sometimes the days coincide, and sometimes they don't. That averages about three to four days of call per week. Hospital call requires me to admit patients to the hospital for the other physicians after hours and troubleshoot problems with inpatients. This sometimes requires me to stay up at the hospital most or all of the night followed by a full day of clinic the next day. This can include responsibilities anywhere from newborns to a patient on a ventilator in the intensive care unit.

My typical workday is ten or eleven hours in the office with an hour scheduled for lunch. However, due to unexpected events, I am sometimes running late, patients show up late for appointments or walk in without an appointment, or someone is just being downright sick and needs a lot of time and attention, I rarely get to eat. I have Wednesday in which no patients are scheduled in the office. That is the day I round at the nursing home or have administrative meetings such as the nursing home, health department, or office. That usually encompasses most if not the entire day. My typical workday starts an hour or so before my first clinic patient at 8:00 a.m. I have to round at the hospital first, review anything that I did the day before that came in, and do paperwork until my first patient. I review and sign somewhere around a hundred orders throughout the day and close to that many documents that enter the system, such as consult notes, reports of diagnostic studies, etc. These include orders from the nursing home or home health agencies, as well as a mountain of forms that must be completed by various entities requiring that I show justification before whichever test or treatment will be authorized. Very frequently I find things such as a stack from the pharmacists from nursing facilities or insurance companies requesting that I write what amounts to an essay justifying why I chose one particular medication or combination of medications over another, or a form that must be completed before a patient can receive a certain home health service or medical equipment.

I have one assistant who does nothing but prepare my paperwork and liaison between the rest of the world and me. It is literally a full-time job. Then quite often during the day I will receive calls from patients who "just want to ask me a few questions." I literally do not have time to stop and answer the phone. That would take away from those patients in my exam room waiting patiently to be seen. Again, no one gets to see the wizard. There is too much other stuff to do.

Once clinic starts it is non-stop patients until the last patient leaves. This is followed by another round at the hospital to tidy up anything that happened during the day. If I am on call my phone will ring almost every twenty minutes or so all night until 7:00 a.m. the next morning. Saturday we have clinic as well, so Saturday morning is the same as any other weekday, except I am usually out of the office by 2:00 p.m. If I am on call during the weekend, I can expect to stay in the hospital pretty much every day until about 7:00 p.m., longer if someone is critically ill.

Oh, at some point in there I have to see my children, do laundry, buy groceries, clean my house, and sleep. Oh, and write this book, but right now it's 2:30 a.m. This is the only free time I have. I don't plan anything further out than two hours away, because there is no guarantee that I won't be tied up somewhere. That makes dinner and a movie impossible. That's three hours.

So no, I am not playing golf. Thanks for asking, though.

Before one thinks that the above discussion amounts to nothing more than whining, it is assuredly not. I like my profession for the most part. I dislike the administrative and legal burdens placed upon me, but I truly enjoy helping others.

# What Will the Future Bring?

I received the following last week:

> Dear Andrew,
>
> I am announcing the closure of my practice in Southern Indiana and Kentucky. Unfortunately, the current economic climate in medicine makes it impossible for me to continue as a solo practitioner. For this reason, my wife and I have made the decision to move out of state to relocate closer to our families. It has been a genuine pleasure and an honor providing for the health and well being of your patients, and it has not been an easy decision for me to give up that privilege.

Also that week.

> It is with heartfelt sadness that I announce that I will be closing my practice... After a lot of thought and prayer over the last year, I feel that this is the decision I must make. It has been impossible for a solo physician practice to survive. We are going the way of the dinosaur. As a solo practitioner, it is difficult anymore to keep up with all the changes in health care, billing, and ever-increasing technology. I've always tried to provide quality care for all of my patients. With the support of my family, my patients have always come before everything else.

I have always recommended to my patients, "You need to take care of yourself first so that you can take care of others." I feel that the time has come that I need to start taking that same advice. My family needs me to be around more as well. I want to be a doctor, wife, mother, daughter, and sister again, not a business owner or manager.

I will miss the patients for whom I have cared for the last twenty-two years. I will also miss the wonderful staff at the hospital with whom I have been blessed to have known and worked with. You will always be in my thoughts. I wish every one of you the best.

Is this the future of health care in America? Some days I wonder if I should have been an electrician like my father, but then I see the faces in the waiting room. I remember the prisoners of war; I remember my shipmates. I see those people right in front of me who need my help, and I see them light up when they see me, because they know I care about them.

My name is Andy, and I am on the front line of medicine.

# Epilogue

Excerpt of a letter to Bubba:

Thank you so much for your hospitality on my recent trip to Anchorage. As you know, it's always been a life-long dream of mine to visit the Last Frontier. It's a shame that I couldn't stay longer, but unfortunately life sometimes gets in the way of living. It's difficult to find the time for myself with my responsibilities at work and everything going on at home with the four children.

I don't know ultimately what will happen here. Sometimes I think I can work things out, especially for the kids' sake, but there are also days that I don't know if that is the right thing to do. Thank you for offering a listening ear. Good friends like you are hard to find.

I especially enjoyed our hike yesterday toward Knik Glacier, so thank you for that. The view was spectacular, and the wildlife that we saw, including the eagle and moose, was amazing. The dust that kicked up as we hiked Jim Creek, though, did remind me an awfully lot of the Middle East, reminiscent of our deployment together as infantry medics in Desert Storm. I kept searching the path for cluster bombs and land mines though. I guess some things just don't fade as quickly as we would hope. I was pleased that I brought my combat boots. I am so grateful that I did not get rid of them after I left the navy.

That experience and training definitely helped as we hiked those fifteen miles yesterday. I suppose being stationed with the marines does have its advantages, and no, I wasn't about to sing a cadence. I still had bagpipe music playing in my head from our visit to the Highlander Games earlier in the day.

You have a beautiful hospital there. Thank you for the tour. I can imagine being a critical care, intensive care nurse in a hospital such as yours can be quite a challenge. I know that, even in my local hospital back home where I'm currently chief of rehab services, treating a critically ill patient can be challenging and stressful. I know when I have a patient in the intensive care unit it adds just another layer of responsibility to my already sometimes-overwhelming situation. I'm glad that, as a family physician in Corydon, I have the luxury of access to specialists with whose expertise I can draw. That's so much different when I was ship's physician in the navy. Being solely responsible for the lives of my crewmembers was quite an experience. Those men and women were truly my friends and family during deployments. I remember once an officer, who was also my good friend, had a stroke while underway, and we were without access to some of the more basic diagnostic tests. I feel the military has definitely honed my skills as a clinician so that I could function reasonably well in any situation.

Your shoulder should heal on its own and won't need surgery. I'm privileged that you allowed me to look at it. Of course without an X-ray it can be difficult to diagnose orthopedic problems, but I'm pretty confident you sustained a grade II AC separation. We were fortunate to find that foreign body under your son's eyelid. He was pretty uncomfortable after sand landed in his eye when we were on top of the butte. Typically foreign bodies like that will get stuck under the upper lid, and it's an easy thing to avert the lid like I did and remove the speck. That typically fixes the problem. I hope everyone begins to feel better soon.

I really enjoy helping others, and I feel that it's my calling to be a family physician. I like the fact that I can help everyone, from delivering babies all the way to old age and eventual death. I do it all.

As I was waiting to board my airplane this morning to go home, I saw a large display on the wall. It was honoring the Alaskan bush pilots. I was absolutely enthralled with them. I couldn't help but relate to them and what they do. Their calling is to help others, often at their own peril. That dedication and commitment is amazing. I wonder, though, even today how do those in the more remote areas seek medical care? What happens when there is an emergency? I couldn't help but think about the time I treated Iraqi prisoners of war during Desert Storm. I had my aid bag, which stored all the medical gear that I thought I would need. I would go from camp to camp and treat those who were wounded or otherwise injured. The language barrier was a problem, but I did learn to adapt. That was an incredible experience. It was one of the most rewarding times of my life.

There are days, especially like now, when I sit and wonder if I am doing what I was meant to do. I am certain that being a physician is part of that. I did not choose the profession—it chose me. I know that. I could not dedicate myself to the long hours, often over a hundred a week, the time away from my family, and the increasing pressures of running a business in which the future is uncertain if it was not what I was meant to do. I am not necessarily unhappy where I am. I am part of a group practice, and our new medical office building is exciting. We are growing, and there is certainly no lack of people here for me to take care of. I enjoy my community, and I enjoy my patients. I am touched when I see a child running through the store that I personally delivered. There is no greater satisfaction.

I just don't know if it is what I was meant to do. Sometimes I feel that I was meant to do something more, something greater with my life. Life is too short to waste waiting for something to happen. My father and my father's father died relatively young. As we all know, genetics plays a large part in our health. Every day at work I see people who are struggling with their health, often due to no one's fault. Often it is their genetics that predisposed them. I frequently see people get diagnosed with terminal illness at an early age. I see it because I am the one who diagnoses it. I have the burden of telling these people that, despite what they do, they will die. That is a difficult thing to face. Both for them and for me. It is difficult for me, because I care. I was once told that I could expect a 50 percent mortality rate as my unit crossed the berm into Iraq. I was nineteen years old. I had to face my mortality. Three days later on my twentieth birthday as I am treating POWs and listening intently to the gunfire around me, my only wish was to live long enough to see the sun set. I got my wish. I feel that now I am on borrowed time. I feel that I must do something with the time I have. I saw my father die, and I want to know that when I die, there will be no question that I did everything in my power to help others and better myself.

Unfortunately, I am trapped. My medical practice, although a wonderful thing that I am very proud of, is also an anvil weighing me down. I am Bob Cratchit chained to the responsibilities of an office building and a medical practice and financial debt that I would have never thought possible in my entire life. Chains of my own doing to be sure, but chains nonetheless. Then there are the children. Is it possible to fulfill my dream and be a good father? I think so. I was proud of you when you followed your dream and packed your family up, moving from Louisville to Willow Creek. You took them with you, and they are better for it.

I guess it doesn't matter anyway. I cannot be freed from my responsibilities here. I cannot magically produce the amount of money it would cost to have the opportunity to walk away. My debt on the building alone is just shy of one million. I am still paying for my medical school debt and have a mortgage payment. Then there's the second mortgage that I took out to originally buy into the practice before we eventually merged with a hospital due to health care reform. So, as I sit here on my airplane and wish to answer my calling, I sadly cannot.

I saw that Bowman Field has Cessna lessons. I wish that I had the time and resources to take them. I would like to do that. I daydream that I could be a bush pilot, just like those men whose stories are on the wall at the airport. I would fly to the remotest parts of Alaska providing medical care to those who need my services. I would, of course, recruit you, my good friend and my confidant, as my assistant and my nurse. Your mechanical abilities would also come in handy in a pinch I would suspect. We have been on many great adventures in the twenty years that I have known you, and I trust you with my life.

You have been my boss, my mentor, and my role model. You are my hero. Thank you for listening.

Andy

To which he replied with this e-mail:

Managed care hasn't really hit out in the villages yet.

Flying lessons are going well.

# Appendix A

## Evaluation and Management Overview

There are three key components when selecting the appropriate level of E/M service provided: history, examination, and medical decision-making. The elements required for each type of history are described below. As the type of history becomes more intensive, the elements required to perform that type of history also increase in intensity. For example, a problem-focused history requires the documentation of the chief complaint (CC) and a brief history of present illness (HPI), while a detailed history requires the documentation of a CC, an extended HPI, plus an extended review of systems (ROS), and pertinent past, family, and/or social history (PFSH).

A CC is a concise statement that describes the symptom, problem, condition, diagnosis, or reason for the patient encounter. The CC is usually stated in the patient's own words. For example, patient complains of upset stomach, aching joints, and fatigue. The medical record should clearly reflect the CC.

HPI is a chronological description of the development of the patient's present illness from the first sign and/or symptom or from the previous encounter to the present. HPI elements are:

- Location (example: left leg);
- Quality (example: aching, burning, radiating pain);
- Severity (example: ten on a scale of one to ten);
- Duration (example: started three days ago);
- Timing (example: constant or comes and goes);
- Context (example: lifted large object at work);
- Modifying factors (example: better when heat is applied); and
- Associated signs and symptoms (example: numbness in toes).

There are two types of HPIs: brief and extended. A brief HPI includes documentation of one to three HPI elements, whereas an extended HPI should describe four or more elements of the present HPI or associated comorbidities or the combination of at least four elements of the present HPI and/or the status of at least three chronic or inactive conditions depending on which guideline one chooses to use.

ROS is an inventory of body systems obtained by asking a series of questions in order to identify signs and/or symptoms that the patient may be experiencing or has experienced. The following systems are recognized for ROS purposes:

- Constitutional Symptoms (e.g., fever, weight loss);
- Eyes;
- Ears, Nose, Mouth, Throat;
- Cardiovascular;
- Respiratory;
- Gastrointestinal;
- Genitourinary;
- Musculoskeletal;
- Integumentary (skin and/or breast);

- Neurological;

- Psychiatric;

- Endocrine;

- Hematologic/Lymphatic; and

- Allergic/Immunologic.

There are three types of ROS: problem pertinent, extended, and complete. A problem pertinent ROS inquires about the system directly related to the problem identified in the HPI, whereas an extended ROS inquires about the system directly related to the problem(s) identified in the HPI and a limited number (two to nine) of additional systems. A complete ROS inquires about the system(s) directly related to the problem(s) identified in the HPI plus all additional (minimum of ten) organ systems. Those systems with positive or pertinent negative responses must be individually documented. For the remaining systems, a notation indicating all other systems are negative is permissible. In the absence of such a notation, at least ten systems must be individually documented.

PFSH consists of a review of three areas: past history including experiences with illnesses, operations, injuries, and treatments; family history including a review of medical events, diseases, and hereditary conditions that may place the patient at risk; and social history including an age appropriate review of past and current activities. The two types of PFSH are pertinent and complete. A pertinent PFSH is a review of the history areas directly related to the problem(s) identified in the HPI. The pertinent PFSH must document at least one item from any of the three history areas. A complete PFSH is a review of two or all three of the areas, depending on the category of E/M service. A complete PFSH requires a review of all three history areas for services that, by their nature, include a comprehensive assessment or reassessment of the patient. A review of two history areas is sufficient for other services.

To make matters worse, there are two versions of the E&M documentation guidelines, a 1995 version and a 1997 version. The most substantial differences between the two versions occur in the examination documentation section. Either version of the documentation guidelines, not a combination of the two, may be used for a patient encounter. Additionally, an auditor may choose whichever version he or she feels fit to use, or I suspect whichever version will result in a greater "overpayment" to physicians, in the case of a RAC audit.

The levels of E&M services are based on four types of examination: problem focused (a limited examination of the affected body area or organ system), expanded problem focused (a limited examination of the affected body area or organ system and any other symptomatic or related body areas), detailed (an extended examination of the affected body area(s) or organ system(s) and any other symptomatic or related body areas), and comprehensive (a general multi-system examination or complete examination of a single organ system). An examination may involve several organ systems or a single organ system. The type and extent of the examination performed is based upon clinical judgment, the patient's history, and nature of the presenting problem(s).

The 1997 documentation guidelines, as an example, describe two types of comprehensive examinations that can be performed during a patient's visit: general multi-system examination and single organ examination. A general multi-system examination involves the examination of one or more organ systems or body areas. These are broken down into problem focused, expanded problem focused, detailed, and comprehensive examinations.

For a multi-organ system examination, a problem focused examination includes performance and documentation of one to five elements identified by a bullet in one or more organ system(s) or body area(s). The expanded problem focused exam includes performance and documentation of at least six elements identified by a bullet in one or more organ system(s) or body area(s).

The detailed examination includes at least six organ systems or body areas. The comprehensive exam includes at least nine organ systems or body areas.

A single organ system examination involves a more extensive examination of a specific organ system. The problem focused exam includes performance and documentation of one to five elements, the expanded problem focused included at least six elements, a detailed exam includes at least twelve elements, and a comprehensive exam includes all elements.

Medical decision making refers to the complexity of establishing a diagnosis and/or selecting a management option, which is determined by considering the following factors: the number of possible diagnoses and/or the number of management options that must be considered; the amount and/or complexity of medical records, diagnostic tests, and/or other information that must be obtained, reviewed, and analyzed; and the risk of significant complications, morbidity, and/or mortality as well as comorbidities associated with the patient's presenting problem(s), the diagnostic procedure(s), and/or the possible management options.

The risk of significant complications, morbidity, and/or mortality is based on the risks associated with the following categories: presenting problem(s); diagnostic procedure(s); and possible management options. The assessment of risk of the presenting problem(s) is based on the risk related to the disease process anticipated between the present encounter and the next encounter. The assessment of risk of selecting diagnostic procedures and management options is based on the risk during and immediately following any procedures or treatment. The highest level of risk in any one category determines the overall risk, and the levels are described as minimal, low, moderate, or high.

Okay, got all that? Me neither.

# Appendix B

This thesis means a lot to me. It is my experiences before, during, and after Desert Storm. It is what I did, how I felt, and how it has changed my life. The making of this thesis started five years ago when I enlisted into the United States Army Reserve at the age of seventeen, and even though the war has been over for two years, I can still feel its aftershocks. This is my story.

Feb. 4, 1991: Today I did something I might regret. I volunteered to go to Saudi Arabia. I really don't know why I did this, but I don't as of yet regret the choice. When the Command Sergeant Major asked for volunteers to go to the theater of action, I just stood up and gave them my name. I don't know why I did this, but I did. Let's hope and pray that I did not make a fatal mistake.

Feb 16: This last week I've been at Fort Jackson, South Carolina. We've been doing things like firing our M-16s, being issued our equipment, and basically doing nothing. Since we last talked, I've gone from contacts to glasses. I hate them, but I don't have a choice. With the blowing sand, it would be impossible to keep them. Tomorrow morning we leave for Saudi. Let's all hope that we'll all be home soon.

Feb. 18, Day 1: We flew all day today. First of all, we went from Jackson to New York. On the way out I saw the Statue of Liberty. That was the last US land I'll be on in a long time.

We then flew from New York to Rome. Here we couldn't leave the plane because the threat of terrorists was too great. So all of Rome I saw was a runway. From Rome we went to where I am now, some obscure air base near Daharan, I think. Actually, I'm not really sure where I am, except that I'm in a desert.

Today I heard some disturbing news. I won't be with the 18th Airborne Corps as was originally planned. I'll be with the 7th Corps, and the 7th Corps is artillery and infantry on the front line. Half of the group from my unit went to the 18th, and the rest went to the 7th Corps. Tomorrow we'll be moving to a point forty-seven miles from the border. I guess I'll see how that turns out later.

Feb. 19-20: I've learned that we are at (have landed at) King Fahd (sp?) airbase. This airbase is not on the map as of yet, since it is not completed. We are approximately forty-five miles or there-abouts east of the country (Bahrain?) out there in the Persian Gulf. Today (20th) we're supposed to move to fifty miles from the border, to a place called Al Quaissmah. As I'm now attached to the 7th Corps, I'll probably be closer to the border before this is all over with.

Feb. 21: After leaving the reception station at King Fahd, we went to the large international airport there and were loaded into a C-130. We flew for an hour due north to a small airport.

This airport was heavily guarded and looked very trashed. We saw a platoon of Brits here. I like their uniforms better.

Once we were unloaded, we were crammed into deuce and a halves and drove approximately twenty miles on asphalt and another thirty on dirt through the desert to the 7th Corps replacement camp.

Feb.22: I lost more of my friends today. Those of us remaining were split into about six smaller groups. I was in the 1st Infantry group, along with about five others. And then there was five.

Well, shit happens. Right now I am twevle miles from the Iraqi border. At night we can hear the artillery bombing. Oh, I almost forgot. I've been assigned to the 1st Infantry Division, 3-37th Armor Battalion. "Looks like I'm in the front line." Anyway, this place is a trip. We sleep in tents with no floors, only sand, and no cot. So, I sleep in the sand. At 5:00 a.m. we have something called "stand to," which means that we get dressed and stand in a foxhole for an hour in the freezing air, with weapons and no ammunition. Oh what fun. They say that if there is going to be an offensive for the other side, it will happen at 5:00 a.m. My group was broken down even further today. My last remaining friend from me reserve unit and I were loaded into a truck and sent to our units. He is going to be 2-16th Infantry and I to the 3-37th Armor. As we were travelling, he asked the driver of the truck about his unit. The driver kinda laughed and told him that they were notorious for shooting at each other, and that we would be getting there soon. Curious, I asked him where my unit was. He shook his head and said, "All the way up."

7:48 p.m.: I've finally reached my unit, 3-37 Armor. Actually, only half of my unit (two tank companies plus headquarters) is 3-37 Armor. The other two companies are infantry from the 2-16th. Apparently, these two units swapped companies. So even though my unit is officially an armor unit, we are as much infantry as the infantry unit. Right now we're about seven miles from the border. Tomorrow I move up to my duty station (platoon?) closer to the front. Tonight I'm spending the night in a track with two tankers. They're pretty cool. I've met my Platoon Sgt. He's laid back. The ground war is supposed to start the 24th, on day before my birthday. Some present, huh? I've finally been separated from the last member of the 5010th USA Hospital. I said good-bye to him today. I guess I'll see him at summer camp. From his unit I was loaded up into the mail truck and driven to my unit. The mail truck was the only vehicle that was going that far north. The rumor is that I'll only be here for 180 days. We'll see…

Feb. 23: Today I found my duty station. They're 3.3 miles from the border. Tomorrow we make the big ground offensive. I'll be in one of the first companies and the first unit from the 7th Corps through the breach in the Iraqi lines. Right now I'm at an aid station, which is in a "track", an armored personnel carrier or APC. Anyway, the British are out here also. Those guys will swap the clothes off your back. Right at this time, I am enjoying a piece of sharp cheese and a corned beef sandwich. We traded some of our stuff for some of their stuff. Tomorrow at 5:00 a.m. we move out.

I learned a few new things today. One is that the M-16 that I was issued at Fort Jackson is useless out here. It is the old A1 model, and everyone out here is using the A2 model. Unfortunately, the A2 ammunition does not work in an A1 rifle, so I exchanged mine for one of theirs. Also, there is a medic out here that is kinda nuts. They say that he snapped and threatened a sergeant. I was told to try to avoid him if I can.

Feb. 24: Today the ground war started. After pulling a four-hour guard shift last night, we woke up at 4:30 a.m. and prepared to leave. We then waited...until 8:30 a.m.. After getting word that we were finally moving out, we climbed onto our track and moved out. We reached what was called a berm. Actually it was a wall of dirt and sand about eight feet high. Our B and C platoons and engineers had already broken down the berm in a few places, so all we had to do was drive on through. Let me explain the strategy as I see it. 3rd Battalion, 37 Armor Brigade would be the spearhead for the entire 7th Corps' attack on Iraq. B and C companies clear the area (a path north), and then the medics (me) and the rest of the corps would follow. It is our job to secure the area for the rest of the US troops. Even though the berm was the border, the Iraqi troops were farther back. We are expecting a 50 percent casualty rate.

We went through the berm, taking no casualties and about 400-600 POWs for the 3-37th alone. We then traveled north to the place where the bunkers were located. They were only about four feet deep, covered with tin with a little dirt on top. Our artillery effectively blew them to hell before we even got there. After breaching the bunkers, we kept traveling north until we reached this place to rest. Tomorrow, we're supposed to travel north some more, securing the area and then, when the 7th Corps moves east toward Kuwait, follow in reserve behind them. We only move during the day, because at night we cannot see the minefields.

Feb. 25: Today is my twentieth birthday. I wonder how Ace and Johnny (the two tankers) are doing. Those two will always be a riot, even if I never see them again. While I was visiting them, all they had to do was play Rummy, since it takes four to play Spades, and clean their weapons. The entire time I was there, all they did was argue about minutia. I guess all that stress, plus being cramped in that track, made them both neurotic.

Today we sit. After traveling for about two hours in an easterly direction, we stopped and waited. Well, we are still waiting. It appears as though we have reached some resistance, as I can hear machine gun fire in front of us. I wonder if I will live to see the sun set today? Here, though, all is quiet for now. Word is that we move at night...

Feb. 26: Today, we are supposed to move north against the Republican Guard, but we changed direction (as British units encounter the guard), and we continue east toward Kuwait.

Feb. 27: We had a rough fifth night of travelling. Late last night we found ourselves about half way to Kuwait. Now, however, we are a mere twelve miles, and still we press on.

Today I see the war in a different light. For the past couple of days, we have been taking prisoners like mad, 20,000 yesterday and 14,000 the day before. It has gotten to be so bad (about the number of prisoners) that we don't even keep guards on them anymore. They come staggering into our convoy half-starved and desperate. We don't even stop, just keep going. Someone else will stop and feed them.

For example, today a group of about twenty to thirty Iraqi soldiers walked into our camp. They were starved and only wanted to be fed. We didn't even bother to load our weapons; we knew they were harmless. They came in half clothed, some without shoes. A lieutenant of ours gave a pair of socks to one soldier whose feet were red and swollen from walking. They walked through our camp, and we all just stared. This is the enemy? What kind of madman would leave his own people to starve? Of course, it didn't help that we blew their supply lines to hell.

Feb. 27. Later that day: "Strange things are afoot at the Circle-K," (to quote the movie *Bill and Ted's Excellent Adventure*). Since 7:00 p.m. I have had the strange duty of being a prisoner guard for on of Hussein's Republican Guard. He had taken some shrapnel in his left upper arm and left side-only superficially, however. One of our sergeants asked if someone would watch him, and I said that I would.

His name is Rashad Sanad (according to he Field Medical Card), and he speaks no English. After a long, tiresome ordeal lasting a few hours, I learned that he had to go to the bathroom. (And that's the way it's been all night. Luckily he sleeps most of the time, only to awaken once in a while to mumble something in Arabic.)

Feb. 28: Today we had a cease-fire. I hope it lasts. I will probably never forget this night as long as I live. We have reached a station in which we are treating one thousand-plus Iraqi soldiers. I have seen personally about three to four hundred. They are nice people, quick to smile and very understanding. Surprisingly, they are glad to see us. I suppose their situation couldn't get any worse.

These people are tired and hungry. Some of them have been walking (and some without shoes) for days and haven't eaten for over four days. Every one of them has blisters on their feet, and some of them are trench-footed.

There is a place we passed about two clicks (kilometers) from here where our bombing has taken out some soldiers. There are bodies everywhere, bits and pieces, decapitation and charring everywhere. All these people want, like all of us soldiers, is to simply go home.

A doctor from another unit was brought to us for some reason. It was unfortunate that he was in a body bag. Apparently the Jeep he was riding in hit a land mine on his side. The chaplain had to go through his pockets to find some identification and an address or phone number so he could reach the man's wife. A group of men surrounded the chaplain as he did this. I didn't bother to look. The idea just didn't appeal to me. The roads are already littered with the dead, and on the way one to one of the prisoner holding areas I have to walk past a ditch where more dead are thrown. At least they are in body bags, but it's still an eerie feeling to walk near them.

March 1: Today we set up an aid station for the POWs. We have moved them into a bottled water plant warehouse. They are burning boxes and crates to keep warm, since most don't have blankets. The engineers are starting to blow up bunkers full of Iraqi weapons. One of these blew up near the warehouse. The Iraqis must have thought that we were bombing them again, because they almost stampeded us trying to get out.

We brought them water. That was a nightmare. They were so thirsty that they were walking over concertina wire in their bare feet to try to get a bottle. It was Evian bottled water, of all things. A few shots were fired over their heads, and they finally settled down.

March 2: Yesterday we travelled north to be at those peace talks at some airfield in Iraq. They say that this is one big dog-and-pony show, especially since Hussein had told his people that we have surrendered to them. The few Republican Guard that are left think they have won, but of course they are wrong.

The POW camp was set up 100 km from Kuwait City in one direction (south) and 3 to 4 km from the Iraqi border in the opposite direction (north). We set up a semi-permanent camp and finally got a chance to take a bath out of a bucket of water and get cleaned up after over a week wearing the same clothes. That type of bath is often called, provided there are no females within earshot, a bitch bath or a whore's bath since, as the story goes; the only areas that a whore really washes are the armpits and the groin area.

March 3: We jumped today. I'm now sitting in some Iraqi town forty miles from Basrah in a town called Safwan. We learned of some of the atrocities the Iraqi army committed. One woman here said that she was lucky that she was poor. They only shot her husband and broke her arm. (She has six kids.) If she was rich, they would have looted her and taken her family as slaves. The story of her goes as follows: The Iraqi army came into her house and demanded that her husband join the army. He refused. They then broke her arm and again demanded that her husband join. He again refused. They then proceeded to rape her in front of him. He refused again. Apparently frustrated, they then killed him and left her. When we arrived, we found the children playing with an unexploded cluster bomb.

Another thing we saw today was a man who came to us who had been a prisoner of war of the Iraqis. They had tortured him by placing electrodes on his ankles. The electricity turned his ankles to mush. The doctor says he will never be able to walk again.

One of our medic tracks was sent to a nearby farm. It appeared as though one of the children was harvesting tomatoes when he stepped on a cluster bomb or land mine. The explosion effectively blew him in half. The little boy died, screaming, while the medics tried to save him. I saw the medic who made the run today. He looked a bit pale and wasn't feeling the best.

March 4: Today we did nothing. We jumped again and now are somewhere in the outskirts of Safwan. We have remained in camp, just relaxing. We are supposed to jump today, but we'll see. It looks to me as if we'll be here for a while.

I met the crazy medic today. Actually, he's kinda nice. He's strange, but nice. I say strange in the sense that his personality clashes with the military. He's too much of a free spirit. I finally learned the true story behind what happened the night that he supposedly snapped. Some sergeant told him that he was supposed to be on guard duty at the M-60 machine gun the night before I arrived. According to the Geneva Convention, as he as well as I see it, medics are noncombatants. This means that they are not allowed to fire on enemy troops unless they threaten the life of one of his patients. Therefore, a medic shouldn't be at watch with a machine gun. He explained this to the sergeant, but it fell on deaf ears. The sergeant left the medic and went back to his tent. The medic followed the sergeant to the tent, and words were exchanged. This heated up tempers until they were in each other's face. The medic then left. The next morning the medic was brought up on charges for disobeying a direct order and disrespecting a noncommissioned officer.

March 6: We're still at camp. This makes day three here. Sometime during this time we heard a sniper shooting behind us in a quarry. Two others and I followed the sound, but apparently we chased off whoever it was. We never heard him since. The place we are camped at is rather unusual. It's very hilly, and embedded in the hills are bunkers stockpiled with ammunition, RPGs, and AK-47s. The engineers are systematically blowing them up one by one. That's fine, but I don't know how close we are to them. The explosion is deafening, even louder than the artillery fire, and the shockwave throws a wave of air on us that almost uproots the stakes keeping down our camouflage nets. One explosion was so close that it rocked our track, which weighs, I think, around twenty tons. In Safwan, one man driving a track was hit in the face by shrapnel from one of the exploding bunkers

It rained last night and all day yesterday. The smoke from the burning oil fields made the rain black and greasy. In some places the oil has accumulated into pools a few inches deep. They say we'll move today, but they say that every day.

Today was a rather special day. We were given a few boxes of fresh oranges. This is the first real food we have had to eat in a long, long time. Up until now we have been eating MREs—

meals, ready to eat. It is essentially all dehydrated food. They are somewhat edible for the first couple of weeks, but after a while eating them becomes torturous. The crazy medic and I, who by now have become pretty good friends, confiscated a box of oranges in an attempt to make orange juice "wine." We squeezed all the juice from the oranges, added sugar, and put it in bottled water jugs. We didn't have balloons, so we improvised and placed condoms over the top to catch the escaping carbon dioxide.

March 10: I'm still here. I broke my headphones in transit from the states to my unit, so I have been without tunes for some time. Luckily someone gave me a pair of headphones today, so I've been listening to music all day. The orange fizz, as I called it, turned out decent. We didn't let it ferment long enough to do any good, but a psychological buzz is just as good as a real one.

There's one old medic here who is quite a tinkerer. Today, his project is kite making. He made one and flew it so high (due to the constant wind out here) that we couldn't see it anymore. The kite was about four feet long with a tail of about ten feet. We really surprised the helicopter pilots who flew by today. They couldn't believe that they were seeing a kite in the sky.

It's spring here. Small white flowers are blooming everywhere. In some places it looks like a carpet of them. They are the only things growing in this sand at the moment. The temperature has stayed cool because of the oil smoke. It hovers about us and blocks out the sun. In some places it is so dark that headlights are needed at noon, and it is still hard to see. Of course, the bad thing about the smoke is that it leaves everything outside, including us, covered in a fine layer of soot.

Since we live in tracks, not all of us can sleep inside it. Therefore, some of us, like myself, sometimes sleep on a cot or litter in the sand. It's strange to wake up in the morning and realize the only thing above the sand is one's head. The scorpions are a problem, too. They are everywhere. I spent many an afternoon tormenting a captured scorpion. Some of them out here are very poisonous.

There is a potentially dangerous foe lurking around our camp. Dogs. They have gotten fierce lately. A lot of them are feeding of the dead Iraqi bodies that litter the roadsides, and it appears that they like the taste. A dead horse was lying on the side of the road when we moved in; now the only thing left is a few bones. The dogs ate the rest. They have gotten so fierce that we have to carry a loaded weapon with us when we head out to find a place to defecate.

Since we are in the front, we do not have such luxuries as running water or any sort of toilet facilities nor the wood to build any. Since there are no females in combat units, we have no problem finding a place to urinate. Actually, anywhere so long as it isn't atop someone's sleeping bag, usually works. It is the other that causes problems. It is a matter of finding a shovel, a roll of toilet paper (which is always in short supply), and heading off behind a sand dune, if one is available. Some people have been known to walk a half mile to find a place isolated enough to squat in peace. Of course, we have to take all of our equipment with us. This includes our weapon, our protective mask, our helmet, sometimes the flak jacket (which weighs about fifteen pounds), and web gear to include: two full two-quart canteens, two full ammo pouches, poncho, and finally the attached shoulder straps. We carry all that just because nature called. But I digress. One of our fuel Hemmit drivers went out "behind a dune" so to speak and was attacked by a wild dog. He had to shoot it. Upon inspection of the surrounding area, it was found that the dog was protecting her puppies. Feeling bad, he took one of the puppies with him, so now we have a puppy roaming among our ranks.

March 13: We moved today. We are now three km from the DMZ or demarcation line. We moved west. At least we have new sand to look at. I saw a shepherd and his flock of sheep and one camel today. Kinda biblical, I thought. He moved them right through our camp. We waved, and he waved back.

March 18: Moved again. Today I used the phones. I was packed into a Hummer with about eight other people, and our lieutenant drove us to the phones. On our way we passed a Red Cross tent hospital. There were refugees swarming all over the place. The roadsides were lined with people looking for a hand-out. Luckily for them, we had leftover MREs, and we "accidentally" dropped them as we passed the hospital. We were told that we should not feed the refugees because they would choke up the roads and start invading our camps looking for food or supplies.

The smoke was very thick along the paved roads. We were so close to some of the oilfields that we could feel the heat from them. The air felt greasy as we passed. Everyone at home was fine, so now I feel better. That was the first contact with the States that I had since I arrived here a month ago. I received no mail, because I didn't receive an address until I reached my duty station, and no mail was being picked up or delivered since we move so much.

March 20: We moved today. They say that we are going to replace the 82nd Airborne near the Euphrates River, near Baghdad. As we progressed northward, we saw harsh desert turn to farming communities, tomatoes mostly. We saw a herd of wild camels as we trekked onward. It was a very strange thing to see. The funniest thing happened to us, though. We got lost. We were so lost, in fact, that we had to ask a shepherd, who was with his flock of sheep in the absolute middle of nowhere, where we were and how to get to where we were going. If he would have been standing at a gas station wearing coveralls with his name embroidered over the breast, the joke would have been complete.

At our last point, we had an Iraqi family as our next-door neighbor. They grew tomatoes and had a flock of sheep. In the morning the wife would come up to us with her children and ask for food. Later in the afternoon, the husband would come with a gas can and ask for gas. They are very friendly people.

March 25: We've been at this new point for three or four days now. Instead of replacing the 82nd Airborne, we are waiting with bated breath whether or not Bush will sign the peace treaty. I really hate this new location. We have moved north and west from Kuwait and are now no longer under the cloud of smoke. Because of this, the sun is pounding down on us. We went from cold mornings and nice evenings to hot, hot, hot. The sun literally drains the strength from me if I ever go out in it. Also, the ground at the particular location is solid rock under a few inches of blowing sand. When nature calls, we must hike for what seems like forever until we find a place where the ground is soft enough to dig into.

Today, we have a new member of our medic crew, a new sergeant However, this sergeant is female. That puts a cramp in our style out here. Now we have to be aware of where we are in relation to her when nature calls. When she first arrived out here, her presence created quite a controversy. Some said that our integrity was compromised because we had to be conscious of not offending her, such as taking a bath out in the open, which we often did, because there was no other place to do it, not to mention the fact that women tend to want some sort of latrine, which could not be quickly constructed or torn apart if we had to move out in a hurry. If we can acquire the material, we are supposed to build a latrine in the next few days. Also, privacy is a big problem, because there isn't any. There is no living quarters other than the vehicles, and not everyone can sleep in them. There is not enough room. However, our sergeant seems to manage well enough out there. The only problem that I saw was that she was prone to taking her baths at night. That in itself is fine. The problem arises where there are bored men roaming the desert with very expensive and very good night vision apparatuses. She might as well have taken it at noon. It would have accomplished the same thing, and she would have been a lot warmer.

If the peace treaty is signed, we get to go south. If not, then we go farther onward into Iraq.

A small bird, the only kind I've seen out here, has found a home in camp. It walks all around us, eating flies and small insects. It stepped on my feet today.

Someone had the presence of mind to bring a horseshoe set out here. That was fun for the first week, but it, along with cards, is becoming very boring. I can only play so many hands of Spades or Euchre or Rummy or whatever before it becomes tedious. We need to move. At least tearing down camp will give us something to do. On our track, a 577, as compared to the smaller 133s which are the "ambulances", we have a small tend extension that folds outward. This then becomes the aid station where a couple of the severely wounded can stay out of the elements. During break-down, we have to dismantle our camouflage netting over us. This is quite time consuming, because the net always gets caught on the equipment stored on the outside of the track. Once the net is rolled up and put away, we tear down the extension and roll it up. It is attached to the top of the track and is tied there. We then store our gear in the track and squirm inside. With all the medical equipment and personal stuff, there isn't much room for us. The whole process takes about an hour.

March 30: Well, we haven't built that latrine yet. On March 29, I was the TC for the female back to her unit, the 201st, and stayed there for the night. That was fine, but I forgot to bring my mask with me, so I couldn't roam the camp. They had running water and showers, but I didn't dare wander too far outside the tent that I was sleeping in for the night. If I would have been caught without my mask, then I could have gotten in some serious trouble, especially since it was at another unit. But, I'm now home, and my error wasn't discovered by anyone who really cared. I now know that I was definitely attached to the wrong unit. The 201st had women. Lots of them. And, since the women wanted equal rights, they are treated exactly as the men are treated. That included sleeping in co-ed tents. That was definitely an odd experience for me. I spent a month and a half without seeing another female, well, American female, and then one day I am sleeping in a tent with ten of them.

They say we'll be out of here in May, so the morale of everyone is way up.

April 15: We finally moved. After packing all day, we finally left this spot and are supposed to head for Camp Hubner in Saudi Arabia. Due to some supposed regulation about activating reservists, I am supposed to be back in the states no later than May fourth. It's about time.

April 16: Yesterday was an experience.

I was asked if I wanted to ride in a fuel Hemmit, since our 577 was so crowded and uncomfortable, and I said yes, so I jumped in the truck with only the minimal of equipment. I left my sleeping bag in the track and only brought enough food with me for the day. We drove from 7:00 a.m. to 6:00 p.m. due south, and I was bounced and tossed around the whole ride. Early in the march, however, my track broke down with major mechanical difficulties, so when we arrived at camp for the night, I had no place to sleep. I begged and borrowed food and a blanket form the other medics for the night. I hope my track shows up soon, because right now I don't know where my luggage is.

I finally got to see everything I missed on the ride up here because I was in a track. Sometime today we are supposed to reach the berm. I now know that we were two days into Iraq. Yesterday we traveled ninety-five miles due south. Today we traveled sixty-five miles due south, reaching the border sometime early in the day and travelling the rest of the way in Saudi.

April 17: We reached Camp Hubner today. Here we start turning in our vehicles and equipment. Of course, now that we are in Saudi, the BS starts up again, like formations and things like that. That's okay, though, because we have showers and hot food here. Best of all is that we're sleeping in tents, and not in the open desert.

I ran into Ace and Johnny. They had a strange tale to tell. When the ground war started, they were left with one broken Bradley Scout Vehicle alone in the desert and didn't have food or water. As a matter of fact, our unit forgot that they were there and didn't send anyone to pick them up when we settled in. On the eighth day out there they finally saw an Apache helicopter and waved at him until he saw them. The chopper pilot then called another unit, and they took them here.

We get to go to a place called Dangertown out here. It's about three miles away, so it's too far to walk. It's really neat. They have a store here, where you can buy stuff, and there are "native crafts" such as prayer rugs and those things that they wear on their heads. Of course, a lot of that stuff is made in another country. There's a food stand here (that's free), as well as a phone center and movie theatre. It's really nice. The entire atmosphere reminds me of a carnival.

April 20: Yesterday I was told, "Pack up. You're supposed to be out of here in forty-eight hours." So now I'm packed and on standby, and I don't know what is going to happen.

Sometime while we were in Iraq, one of our medics was sent home to Ohio. The day he arrived, the town had a parade in his honor. That night he was killed in an automobile accident. We had a funeral service for him here. The entire unit was brought to formation, and the battalion and brigade commanders said a few things. After they were finished, our platoon sergeant called roll call for the medic platoon. We all said, "Here, Sergeant." The last name on the roll call was the dead man, and it was called three times without a response.

April 26: Those forty-eight hours turned out to be four to eight days. That morning, I woke up and left, saying good-bye to everyone, even though they thought I was CID. That was a real pain. Since I mysteriously appeared just before the ground war, claiming to be a reservist, they automatically think I am from the Central Intelligence Division. Of course, the CID does things like that, or so I'm told. Anyway, I was effectively ostracized the whole time I was here, so I don't feel any lost love for most of these people.

I'm at Brigade, and they lost the plane that I was supposed to go home on. So now they have to find another one and find a place for me on that one. I guess I'll see what happens soon. I found my reservist buddy from back home. He was the last person from my unit that I saw, and he was the first person I met on the way back.

April 29: Finally reached the States—in New York at 5:00 a.m. EST.

May 1: I've spent the last few days out processing here at Fort Jackson. We have a lot of down time, which is good so we can wind down.

I guess it's time to try to return to a normal life, whatever that is.

* * *

My name is Andy Morton. I enlisted into the United States Army Reserve on 29 February 1988. At the time, I was a junior in high school. Because I was still in school, I went through basic training during the summer after my junior year. I then when through AIT (advanced individual training) at Fort Sam Houston, Texas as a 91A10-Medical Specialist, often called combat medic, during the summer of 1989.

I did not join the army because I was patriotic; although I am. I did not join because I really needed the discipline; although it helped. I did not join because I needed the adventure, because my life is one big adventure without having to search for it. I joined for only one reason. I joined for the college money.

I chose to be a medical specialist for a variety of reasons. One of which is that the course was short enough to take during the summer. Another is that I was thinking about taking pre-med courses and applying to medical school. At that point, I really had no experience with the medical profession, other than the rare visit to the doctor's office for the flu. No one in my family is a doctor nor even in the health care field. I thought that I needed a little contact with the field before making a choice, so I decided to be a medic. I would be gaining medical experience and be able to pay for school at the same time.

I graduated with honors from AIT and developed a passion for the medical profession. I worked at a nursing home for a few months during my freshman year, but due to lack of time and sleep, I had to quit and concentrate on school. During the summer of 1990, I worked as an emergency room technician at a hospital close to where I grew up. It was there that I really decided that I wanted to be a doctor. During my drill weekends for the reserves, I work on the surgical ward at the Louisville VA hospital. There, too, I find what I do rewarding, even though traveling from Muncie to Louisville once a month is very inconvenient.

In the autumn of 1990, Iraq invaded Kuwait. On January 26, 1991, about 9:00 a.m. on a Saturday morning, I received a telephone call that would change my life forever. At the time, I was here at Ball State in the second semester of my junior year. I had been in class for about a month. The call started by saying, "You are hereby ordered to active duty in support of Desert Storm." I would report to Fort Knox on February 1. Approximately three weeks later, I was in a foreign country wondering how close to the front I was going to end up. Unfortunately, I went all the way.

For me, this was a traumatic change. First of all, I was thrown from a liberal college campus setting into a very disciplined, rigidly structured organization with very little time to adjust. Secondly, I was put in a combat unit. Thirdly, I was alone. I was not a happy camper.

I had a very rough time the first few weeks I was there. In the military's overwhelming brilliance, the sent a reservist with absolutely no field experience to an armored infantry unit on the frontline the day before the offensive. During drill, I usually work at the Louisville VA hospital on the surgical ward. While there I work as a corpsman, which is roughly equivalent to a nursing assistant. I take care of old, sick veterans. I wash them up, change their dressings, take their vital signs, occasionally start an IV, and mostly joke with them (provided they are conscious) until it is time to go home for the weekend and do it again the next month. The only field experience I have received since I graduated from basic is walking from my car to the hospital and back, which is every bit of forty yards or so. Of course, sometimes it is cold or raining, but essentially it isn't very taxing on me.

However, within a span of a couple of weeks, I had been literally dumped into a combat unit in the field. Now only was it a combat unit, it was an armored combat unit in the middle of the war. I was, needless to say, clueless. The first day that I got to my unit, I was directed toward a group of odd box-shaped vehicles on tracks and was told to go jump into that 113 until the 577 could come pick me up.

My reaction was: "Huh?"

They said, "Do you see that deuce and a half?"

"You mean that big truck?"

"Yeah. Now, do you see the Bradley behind that?"

"The what?"

"The tank-looking thing."

"Oh, that."

"Well, directly to the left of that is a small armored vehicle. That is a 113. A 577 is like that, only it has a larger top on it. Got it?"

"Sort of."

Of course that isn't exactly the conversation, but it was very similar to that. It got even worse later on, when we had to put up the camo netting, build a hasty fighting position, put up the tent extension, set up the medical supplies, or basically do anything. I was totally lost.

The transition from civilian to combat-ready soldier was also a mess. Without my book bag slung over my shoulder, I felt very awkward. I couldn't sleep in and skip the war if I wanted to. I was sleeping in the sand with the scorpions, not in my bed or any bed for that matter. During my first few days there, we moved constantly, so we were forced to sit on the track as it pressed onward, broken only by the occasional pop of an anti-personnel mine as it exploded underneath us.

The transformation from civilian to combat-ready soldier, such as the one I experienced, was a very difficult one. The change was literally an adaption from one society to another, completely different one. The rules were different, the lifestyle was different, the norms and values were different. For me, it was a transformation of personality. Expectations of me were different. I was supposed to know a certain amount of medical knowledge, and this knowledge, or lack of, might mean the difference between life and death for some of those men. I have training equivalent to a civilian emergency medical technician, but I had no experience with most of medications that we had, and that was a major part of the job. I had no knowledge of a lot of what I was expected to know out there, because I was never exposed to it—ever. It was not taught at AIT, and I did not learn it during drill weekends. As a student (biology/pre-med) I was not exposed to anything "medical," only basic biology and chemistry stuff. Out there, if they were shot or otherwise wounded, I could help, but if they were sick, then I was completely useless.

Also, I had to adapt to basic lifestyle changes. To go for days without some sort of bath was the norm out there, while here it is regarded as disgusting.

Sleeping in the sand was common, and to be able to sleep on a cot was considered a luxury. Voiding/defecating was pretty much where you felt like it, as long as the smell didn't blow downwind of the vehicle. Defecating without the luxury of a toilet or anything to sit on or even lean on is quite an experience. Dig a hole and try it someday if you think it is easy.

For me, there were very little support mechanisms. Whatever I experienced, I experienced alone. I was the only one from my reserve unit that was assignment to that unit. As a matter of fact, they weren't expecting me when I arrived. I was a complete surprise to them, and of course, they had not made such provisions as finding for me a place to sleep or even a vehicle to ride in. The regulars out there really didn't like me. I was a stranger. I didn't know a damn thing, and I had a lot of luggage. Those soldiers around my own age already had established clicks, of which I was not invited. By the first of April, there was a rumor that I was from the Central Intelligence Division, or CID. They were supposedly known to do things like drop their people off in a unit at awkward times to see if they do anything illegal like keep foreign weapons. Oddly enough, I had not even heard of the Central Intelligence Division until I was accused of being in it! Needless to say, I was pretty much ostracized from that group. The older soldiers did not believe it, but they too had their clicks. They shared different interests than I did, and so I really did not connect with any of them. Essentially, I was alone.

It's a very odd feeling to be thrown into a situation in which literally everything is different. The climate was different, the people, the plants, the animals, everything. Even the stars seemed akilter somehow. They were definitely brighter out there, since the sky was so clear (when the oil smoke didn't blow over us). I remember one particular clear night where a few of us were sitting around just admiring the stars at night. That night was very quiet, at least until a heated argument broke out as to the exact location of the Big Dipper. I had borrowed a pair of binoculars that one of the men had found in a headquarters building in Safwan and was looking at the moon. The sky was so clear that I could actually get a good look at the moon's craters. That's quite different from Muncie's nights, where to be able to even see the moon at night is almost a miracle.

I guess perhaps the clear sky and the dry air were the only things that I really liked out there. I really liked the dry air. Living in the Ohio Valley all my life, I could not believe it when my sinuses cleared up for the first time. However, that's not worth the scorpions, the heat, the sand, and the flies.

The only ties I had to the life that I left were the things I had brought with me. These included a few pictures, everything that was in my wallet, a few civilian clothes, and the headphones and cassette tapes that I bought in Jackson the day before I shipped out. I had no way of contacting friends and family back home for over a month after I got there. I did not have an address to give to them so that they could write me until after the ground war was over. It took about a week after the offensive was over before mail started filtering through to us. Of course, I would not get any of it for a long time. From the time that I sent out a letter until the time that someone received it here at the States was about three to four weeks. It only took eight days to receive a letter, so that was over a month from the time that I sent a letter until I received one. The first contact that I had with anyone from home was on March 18, the first time that I got to use the phone. It was not for another week or so after that before I got my first letter.

Things were so different over there for me that after a while I had trouble remembering what life was like at home. It all seemed like some movie that I saw a long time ago, like none of it was reality. Perhaps this was a way that I could cope with the utter strangeness of it all. I don't know. I would dream of the States, and it was not my life. It was something else that I may or may not have experienced once. I was isolated there, and I had no contact with the "real" world. After a while, I stopped dreaming of home.

That may sound a little farfetched, but it's the truth. Not everyone experienced the same things over there, nor reacted the same way to the war, and I'm sure that no one experienced what I did. The diary only tells what I saw. It doesn't tell what I felt. It doesn't tell about the constant badgering that I received out there from certain members of that unit, because I was a reservist, because I was new. It doesn't fully describe the knot in my stomach every time an explosion would rattle our track. It also doesn't describe the annoyance (frustration?) that I would feel when I would wake up and realize that I was still there, and still alone.

When I returned, I suffered from post-traumatic stress disorder, or PTSD. For about four months after returning to the Midwest from the desert, I suffered from depression, anxiety, weight gain, restlessness, and I was easily startled, especially when I heard sounds that reminded me of explosions or gunfire. Anxiety attacks were the normal rather than the unusual. One doesn't have to be in a war, however, to experience PTSD. It can be experienced by anyone who has had some sort of traumatic experience; the military just put a name to it. For example, if someone was in a car accident and was having problem coping with it—having nightmares or anxiety attacks whenever they ride in a car—it's essentially the same thing.

Here again, I was to go through another transition. One would think that the return trip would be easier, and yet in reality it is a hundred times harder. Why was the return trip so difficult? That is a question that I am still asking myself. I think it is because I expected life to return to "normal" when I came home. Perhaps I thought that the world that I left would be the same one that I was returning to. However, that was not the case. I was not the same person when I returned, nor were they the same people that I left. Everyone was a stranger, and it took time to get reacquainted. Also, not only were the people different, the world in general was not the same one that I left. Life continued while I was gone, and I missed part of it. Even now, someone will make a reference to something that happened during that time, and I have to remind him or her that I wasn't here then. The phase around my house is "it happened when you were gone," like I blinked into nonexistence for three months or something.

Another symptom of PTSD is the constant reliving of the experience. I had a very hard time trying not to think about the desert. Dreams of the war were common, which made it even harder to try to find this life when I was still living the other one. Eventually, though, they faded away, and now I only dream about it once in a great while.

How did I cope once I returned? Oddly enough, I don't think I really did. I think that I just kept at it long enough, and things worked themselves out. There was not much that I could really do; I just survived until I could get a handle on things. I think that I was very fortunate to get home in time for summer vacation. I spent the entire summer thinking. I thought about what I had just gone through and what I was going to do now that it was over.

Once school started that fall, I was still a little wobbly about some things, like my relationship with my girlfriend, and definitely touchy whenever someone mentioned the war, especially during drill weekends. Whenever a group of desert vets got together, the topic invariable would turn to the war. It still happens, two years later; it seems like each one tries to outdo the others in his or her stories, whether it be of fun times spent in Kuwait City or the hardships endured in the desert. Personally, whenever they start mentioning the desert, I just feel sick. I would prefer to get on with my life and let the experience fade into hazy memories where they belong.

The experience wasn't completely a negative one, though. I did bring home some very neat souvenirs. I have two Iraqi gas masks, an Iraqi flag that I found in a headquarters building in Safwan, quite a few of those pamphlets that we dropped on the Iraqis telling than to surrender, a canteen, a complete Iraqi uniform (again from the headquarters building), and an Iraqi license plate that I took off of a burned-out car (an American car, no less) that was in the road.

Also, I don't think I have ever been as emotionally touched as when I shook hands with my father when I came home, and I saw the pride in his eyes. At that moment, I probably felt closer to him than I ever have in my life.

Now, it's two years later. The experience has definitely altered me. I think that now I have a greater awareness and definition of myself. While I was out there, I had plenty of time to analyze my life, and myself. I learned a lot about myself out there. I know myself, and that is something that a lot of us will never really achieve.

During those first few days, I did not know whether or nor I was going to live or die any time soon. That is a disturbing thing to think about. Also disturbing is why I was out there in the first place. Was it for democracy or for national security? Hell no, I was there to protect our oil interests, pure and simple. I was out there risking my life so that we could keep gas prices down. At the time, I thought that my uniform should have had Property of OPEC rather than US Army. What a cause I was willing to die for!

I'm sure that we all think about death every once in a while—I know I have—but to really be confronted with it is something else entirely. To actually wonder if this is going to be the last day on earth is frightening. But I did gain something from the experience. I confronted my own morality, and I have come to terms with it. I became comfortable with the idea that I am mortal. I will eventually die like the rest of us. How would I spend the day if I knew that it was the last day of my life? I wouldn't change a thing. What I am doing now is what I would want to be doing if I were to die tomorrow (except perhaps not sit here all day typing). I am doing what I want to do.

I'm also much more patient and tolerant now than I was before I left. There are very little things now that upset me. Why? Probably because I can now look at them in perspective. The trials and tribulations that we all face each and every day are nothing compared to the trials and tribulations that I faced in the desert.

Another big change for me is my greater appreciation of nature. The natural world is something that we miss here in America because we live in an antiseptic, sequestered life as far away from nature as we can possibly get. We wake up in a climate-controlled house that is more or less animal free, we get in a car that is the same, and we usually work in a place that is not nature. Even when we "go out to nature," it really isn't natural, but a facsimile of it. State parks and forests, provided that we go to them at all, have been altered for our recreation enjoyment. There are roads leading directly to a camping spot where we pitch a tent to keep out of the elements; we even bring with us most of the comforts of home, half of which we don't really need. All we essentially do is move the house to a different location for a few days. Most places have bathroom facilities at our fingertips, and God forbid if there's no toilet paper!

We rush too much in America. Everything is on a timetable. We even have to plan when to relax—and dare not relax any longer than that or we will be late for something. We're also bombarded with too much external stimuli. How can we even take time out with so much floating past us, demanding our attention? When I was in the desert, the land and the people had remained essentially unchanged for centuries. Sure, some of the Bedouins drove Mitsubishi trucks instead of rode camels, but some of them did have camel herds. Out there, there was no real timetable. Most of the time here, we rush and don't even realize it. Out there, all the days were the same, differing only with the passing seasons. Those people did not rush, because there was no reason to.

The sheer enormity of nature out there was overwhelming. As far as the eye could see—which was pretty damn far, because it was completely flat out there, and there was no trees to create an artificial horizon—was nothing but nature, nothing man-made at all. That's quite a change from Indiana. I spent the greater portion of two months surrounded by nature. I lived in it. It was actually very beautiful (as long as we weren't in a part of the country where the actual fighting took place).

On the down side, though, were there any long-term problems caused form the war? That's something that I'm still thinking about and something that I may never have an answer to. The biggest concern that I have is whether or not the smoke form the oil fires affected me in a way that might not turn up for another ten years or so. Also, I know that even now I cannot donate blood until 1994 because I had to take malaria tablets and other, equally nasty stuff. I guess the jury's still out on this, and I won't know unless something happens. I can guess that I didn't contract some exotic parasite, because something like that would have been apparent by now, I hope.

One is whether in general, this experience was a good one or a bad one. I think that it had both qualities. On the short term, the experience itself was very unpleasant, and the initial homecoming not much better. However, as I get further and further in time from the actual event, I increasingly feel that there are some things that I gained from this experience. I am a much stronger person for having done what I did, and I am, in a way, happier because I did it. I really have little doubt in my mind as to what I want to do with the rest of my life, and that allows me to be more focused in what I do. I can concentrate on what I am doing without having that nagging little voice whispering in my ear, asking me if I am really happy doing this.

The second question is, if I had to do this again, would I have volunteered to go? That's a good one. When I initially made the decision, I was really thinking about the men with wives and children that they would have to leave. I really don't know what I would do if I had to decide again. I do know, however, that I don't regret the decision. At the time, I thought that it was the correct one to make.

Now that it is over, what am I doing with myself? Well, I took my medical school entrance exams the following spring after I returned and did well enough to get into IU Medical School. Since I was a semester behind, I had to take extra classes to catch up, taking nineteen hours last semester and finishing up this semester with a grand total of twenty-one. Luckily, though, I'm doing well and plan to graduate this May. After that, it's off to medical school.

And so life goes on.

# Endnotes

1   John Southwick, *Definition of a Profession*, April 1997,http://www.accc.gov.au/content/index.phtml/itemId/277772.

2   Dictionary.com, *Job*, November 17, 2012, http://dictionary.reference.com/browse/job?s=t.

3   Seabury S, Lakdawalla D, Chandra A. Jena AB, "Malpractice Risk According to Physician Specialty," *New England Journal of Medicine* 365, no. 7 (August 2011): 629-36.

4   Federal Highway Administration, *U.S. Population Living in Urban vs. Rural Areas*, May 6, 2011, http://www.fhwa.dot.gov/planning/census_issues/archives/metropolitan_planning/cps2k.cfm.

5   Sara C Charles, "Coping with a Medical Malpractice Suit," *wjm*, January 2001, www.ewjm.com.

6   Hara Estroff Marano, *Laughter: The Best Medicine*, June 21, 2005, http://www.psychologytoday.com/articles/200504/laughter-the-best-medicine.

7   Ph.D., Erin N. Chapman, M.S., Christopher W. Rainwater, M.S., Luis L. Cabo, M.S., and Susan

M.T. Myster, Ph.D Steven A. Symes, "Knife and Saw Toolmark Analysis in Bone: A Manual Designed for the Examination of Criminal Mutilation and Dismemberment," *crime-scene-investigator.net*, December 2010, http://www.crime-scene-investigator. net/KnifeAndSawToolmarkAnalysisInBone.pdf.

8    Derrick J. Pounder, "Postmortem Changes and Time of Death," *dundee.ac.uk*, 1995, http://www.dundee.ac.uk/ forensicmedicine/notes/timedeath.pdf.

9    Deepu G Mathew, Pradeesh Sathyan, and Geetha Vargheese Isaac Joseph, "The Use of Insects in Forensic Investigations: An Overview on the Scope of Forensic Entomology," *Journal of Forensic Dental Sciences* 3, no. 2 (2011): 89–91.

10   *Dalai Lama Quotes*, 2012, http://www.brainyquote.com/ quotes/quotes/d/dalailama158917.html.

11   History of Medicine Division, National Library of Medicine, *The Hippocratic Oath*, February 7, 2012, http:// www.nlm.nih.gov/hmd/greek/greek_oath.html.

12   *Primum Non Nocere*, 2012, http://medical-dictionary. thefreedictionary.com/Primum+Non+Nocere.

13   *History of Copyright Law*, November 10, 2012, http:// en.wikipedia.org/wiki/History_of_copyright_law.

14   Jennifer Medina, *Jackson's Doctor Is Sentenced to Four Years*, November29,2011,http://www.nytimes.com/2011/11/30/ us/michael-jacksons-doctor-sentenced-to-four-years. html?_r=2&adxnnl=1&adxnnlx=1346898879-fewI-JLkVw4Up04vVhLSgDQ&.

15   Leonard Berlin Ronald L. Eisenberg, "When Does Malpractice Become Manslaughter?," *American Journal of Roentgenology* 179, no. 2 (August 2012): 331-335.

16      National Heart Lung and Blood Institute, *What Are Coronary Heart Disease Risk Factors?*, February 1, 2011, http://www.nhlbi.nih.gov/health/health-topics/topics/hd/.

17      American Academy of Family Physicians, *Pay-For-Performance*, 2012, http://www.aafp.org/online/en/home/policy/policies/p/payforperformance.html.

18      *Pay for Performance (Health care)*, May 23, 2012, http://en.wikipedia.org/wiki/Pay_for_performance_(health care).

19      *Pay for Performance (Health care)*, May 23, 2012, http://en.wikipedia.org/wiki/Pay_for_performance_(health care).

20      American Academy of Family Physicians, *Pay-For-Performance*, 2012, http://www.aafp.org/online/en/home/policy/policies/p/payforperformance.html.

21      Michael J Saks, "Medical Malpractice: Facing Real Problems and Finding Real Solutions," *William and Mary Law Review*, 1994: 1-35.

22      Lili Blume, *Are we Really Living Longer? A Closer Look at Life Expectancy Averages.*, February 11, 2011, http://www.neuronalstimuli.com/2011/02/are-we-really-living-longer-a-closer-look-at-life-expectancy-averages/.

23      Morbidity and Mortality Weekly Report, *Ten Great Public Health Achievements — United States, 1900-1999*, April 1, 1999, http://www.cdc.gov/mmwr/preview/mmwrhtml/00056796.htm.

24      Ruth Rendon, "Dentist's Offer to Lower Bill Yields Prostitution Charge," *Houston Chronicle*, August 20, 2004.

25    CNN wire staff, *Pediatrician Ordered to Spend Life in Prison for Molesting Patients*, August 26, 2011.

26    U.S. Department of Health & Human Services, *Summary of the HIPAA Privacy Rule*, 2012, http://www.hhs.gov/ocr/privacy/hipaa/understanding/summary/index.html.

27    Legal Information Institute, *Roe v. Wade*, 2012, http://www.law.cornell.edu/supct/html/historics/USSC_CR_0410_0113_ZS.html.

28    Death Penalty Information Center, *Lethal Injection*, 2012, http://www.deathpenaltyinfo.org/lethal-injection-moratorium-executions-ends-after-supreme-court-decision.

29    Keith Schneider, "Dr. Jack Kevorkian Dies at 83; A Doctor Who Helped End Lives," *New York Times*, June 3, 2011.

30    Today's Military, *ASVAB Test*, 2012, http://www.todaysmilitary.com/before-serving-in-the-military/asvab-test?campaign_id=SEM2012:on:google:ASVAB_MEPS-what_is_the_asvab:Broad.

31    University of Louisville School of Medicine, *Medschool Admissions*, 2008, http://louisville.edu/medschool/admissions/application-process/pre-med-requirements.html.

32    Hollis Turnham, "OBRA '87 Summary," *ncmust.com*, January 23, 2002, http://www.ncmust.com/doclib/OBRA87summary.pdf.

33    Association of American Medical Colleges, *Medical College Admission Test (MCAT)*, 2012, https://www.aamc.org/students/applying/mcat/.

34    Æsop, *Æsop's fables, retold by Joseph Jacobs* (New York: P.F. Collier & Son, 1909–14).

35    Lois A. Wessel, "Nurse Practitioners in Community Health Settings Today," *http://clinicians.org*, February 4, 2005, http://clinicians.org/images/upload/wessel_nurse_practitioners.pdf.

36    American Academy of Family Physicians, "Family Physician and Nurse Practitioner Training," *aafp.org*, October 27, 2010, http://www.aafp.org/online/etc/medialib/aafp_org/documents/press/nurse-practicioners/np-training.Par.0001.File.tmp/NP_Info_FP-NPTraining-Compare-4pgs.pdf.

37    The Free Dictionary, *Allopathy*, 2012, http://medical-dictionary.thefreedictionary.com/allopathy.

38    American Association of Colleges of Osteopathic Medicine, *What Is Osteopathic Medicine?* , 2012, http://www.aacom.org/about/osteomed/pages/default.aspx.

39    Daniel Weiss, *AMA Opposes Giving Pharmacists Prescription Authority*, July 10, 2012, http://www.pharmacytimes.com/news/AMA-Opposes-Giving-Pharmacists-Prescription-Authority.

40    Mel E Jerbert, G Scott Brewster and Mary Lanctot-Herbert, "Ten percent of patients who are allergic to penicillin will have serious reactions if exposed to cephalosporins," *Western Journal of Medicine*, 2000: 341.

41    Justin Kruger and David Dunning, "Unskilled and Unaware of It: How Difficulties in Recognizing One's Own," *Journal of Personality and Social Psychology*, 1999: 1121-1134.

42    *Dunning–Krugereffect,*October31,2012,http://en.wikipedia.org/wiki/Dunning%E2%80%93Kruger_effect.

43    H Admi, Tzuschinsky O, Herer P and Lavis P, "Shift work in nursing: Is it really a risk factor for nurses' health and patients' safety?," *Nurse Econ*, July-August 2008.

44      Fiona Godlee, Jane Smith and Harvey Marcovitch, "Wakefield's Article Linking MMR Vaccine and Autism was Fraudulent," *BMJ,* January 2011.

45      John Thomas, ""Paranoia Strikes Deep": MMR Vaccine and Autism," *Psychiatric Times* 27, no. 3 (2010).

46      Leah Sirkus, Susan Lukacs and Amy Branum, *NCHS Data on Pertussis Hospitalizations in Young Children,* January 7, 2010, http://www.cdc.gov/nchs/data/hestat/pertussis/pertussis.htm.

47      Centers for Disease Control and Prevention , *Pertussis (Whooping Cough),* November 15, 2012, http://www.cdc.gov/pertussis/outbreaks.html.

48      Centers for Disease Control and Prevention, *Vaccines for Children Program (VFC),* August 31, 2012, http://www.cdc.gov/vaccines/programs/vfc/parents/qa-detailed.html.

49      Harvard Health Publications, *Coffee Health Risks: For the moderate drinker, coffee is safe says Harvard Women's Health Watch,* August 2004, http://www.health.harvard.edu/press_releases/coffee_health_risk.

50      David J. Hanson, *Alcohol Problems and Solutions,* 2012, http://www2.potsdam.edu/hansondj/AlcoholAndHealth.html.

51      *Caffeine Side Effects,* 2012, http://www.drugs.com/sfx/caffeine-side-effects.html.

52      American Cancer Society, *What are the Key Statistics About Breast Cancer?,* October 31, 2012, http://www.cancer.org/cancer/breastcancer/detailedguide/breast-cancer-key-statistics.

53      National Cholesterol Education Program, *Risk Assessment Tool for Estimating Your 10-year Risk of Having a Heart*

*Attack*, 2012, http://hp2010.nhlbihin.net/atpiii/calcula-tor.asp.

54      National Heart Lung and Blood Institute, *What Are the Signs and Symptoms of Bronchitis?*, May 1, 2009, http://www.nhlbi.nih.gov/health/health-topics/topics/brnchi/signs.html.

55      National Heart Lung and Blood Institute, *What Are the Signs and Symptoms of Pneumonia?*, March 1, 2011, http://www.nhlbi.nih.gov/health/health-topics/topics/pnu/signs.html.

56      Jennifer Le, "Therapeutic Management of Bronchitis," *American Journal of Managed Care* 11, no. 1 (February 2005).

57      EJ Emanuel, "Cost Savings at the End of Life. What do the Data Show?," *Journal of the American Medical Association* 275, no. 24 (June 1996): 1907-14.

58      IMDb, *Logan's Run*, 2012, http://www.imdb.com/title/tt0074812/.

59      *Post Hoc, Propter Hoc–"After the Fact, Therefore Because of the Fact"* , August 7, 2000, http://www.drury.edu/ess/logic/informal/Post_Hoc__Ergo_Propter.html.

60      Debbie Lawlor, George Davey Smith and Shah Ebrahim, "Commentary: The hormone replacement–coronary heart disease conundrum: is this the death of observational epidemiology?," *International Journal of Epidemiology* 33, no. 3 (2004): 464-467.

61      *U.S. Health Care Costs*, 2012, http://www.kaiseredu.org/issue-modules/us-health-care-costs/background-brief.aspx.

62      Charlie Papazian, *The Complete Joy of Homebrewing* (New York: HarperCollins, 2003).

63      Robert Kazel, *Do you Tend to Undercode? You're Not Alone*, November 22/24, 2004, http://www.ama-assn. org/amednews/2004/11/22/bil21122.htm.

64      William J PhD Rudman, John S Eberhardt III, William Pierce RHIA and Susan, PhD Hart-Hester, *Health care Fraud and Abuse*, September 29, 2009, http://perspectives.ahima.org/health care-fraud-and-abuse/.

65      Patricia A. Dailey, "JCAHO "Forbidden" Abbreviations," *csahq.org*, January 9, 2004, http://www.csahq.org/pdf/bulletin/issue_3/dailey.pdf.

66      U.S. Food and Drug Administration, *FDA and ISMP Launch Campaign to Reduce Medication Mistakes Caused by Unclear Medical Abbreviations*, June 18, 2009, http://www.fda.gov/NewsEvents/Newsroom/PressAnnouncements/2006/ucm108671.htm.

67      Centers for Medicare and Medicaid Services, *Acronym List*, 2012, http://www.cms.gov/apps/acronyms/listall. asp?Letter=ALL.

68      Ross Koppel, "What do we Know about Medication Errors Made via a CPOE System Versus Those Made via Handwritten Orders?," *Critical Care* 9, no. 5 (August 2005): 427–428.

69      Kurt Vonnegut, *Harrison Bergeron*, 2012, http://www.enotes.com/harrison-bergeron/summary.

70      P.L.224-2003, SEC.83, *Information Maintained by the Office of Code Revision Indiana Legislative Services Agency*, http://www.in.gov/legislative/ic/2004/title12/ar15/ch14.5.html.

71      Sarah Kliff, *The Average Employer Health Plan Now Costs $15,745, and that's Kind of Good News*, September 11, 2012, http://www.washingtonpost.com/blogs/wonk-

blog/wp/2012/09/11/the-average-employer-health-plan-now-costs-15980-and-thats-kind-of-good-news/.

72    Centers for Medicare & Medicaid Services, *Physician Self Referral*, March 27, 2012, http://www.cms.gov/Medicare/Fraud-and-Abuse/PhysicianSelfReferral/index.html.

73    Illinois Insurance News, *BCBSIL Parent Company's CEO Pay Increase 61% to $12.9 million*, May 15, 2012, http://www.ilhealthagents.com/blog/tag/health-insurance-company-ceo-salaries-2011/#.ULE2_oYhQZY.

74    Caleb Johnson, *Church and Religion*, 2012, http://www.mayflowerhistory.com/History/plymoth7.php.

75    123HelpMe.com, *Anarchy*, November 24, 2012, http://www.123helpme.com/view.asp?id=39741.

76    William J PhD Rudman, John S Eberhardt III, William Pierce RHIA and Susan, PhD Hart-Hester, *Health care Fraud and Abuse*, September 29, 2009, http://perspectives.ahima.org/health care-fraud-and-abuse/.

77    Laura Joszt, "Top 10 Peeves Doctors Have About Patients," *Physician's Money Digest*, February 22, 2012.

78    Charlie Goldberg, *A Practical Guide to Clinical Medicine*, 2009, http://meded.ucsd.edu/clinicalmed/history.htm.

79    Albert Mehrabian, *Silent Messages: Implicit Communication of Emotions and Attitudes* (Belmont, CA: Wadsworth, 1981).

80    Meredith Levine, "Tell the Doctor All Your Problems, but Keep it to Less than a Minute," *The New York Times*, June 1, 2004.

81    Daniel Levinson, *Testimony on Preventing Health Care Fraud: New Tools and Approaches to Combat Old*

*Challenges*, March 2, 2011, http://www.hhs.gov/asl/testify/2011/03/t20110302i.html.

82    William J PhD Rudman, John S Eberhardt III, William Pierce RHIA and Susan, PhD Hart-Hester, *Health care Fraud and Abuse*, September 29, 2009, http://perspectives.ahima.org/health care-fraud-and-abuse/.

83    Office of Inspector General, Department of Health and Human Services, "Audit of Selected States' Medicaid Payments for Services Claimed To Have Been Provided to Deceased Beneficiaries," *oig.hhs.gov*, September 26, 2006, https://oig.hhs.gov/oas/reports/region5/50500030.htm.

84    William J PhD Rudman, John S Eberhardt III, William Pierce RHIA and Susan, PhD Hart-Hester, *Health care Fraud and Abuse*, September 29, 2009, http://perspectives.ahima.org/health care-fraud-and-abuse/.

85    U.S. Department of Health & Human Services, *HITECH Act Enforcement Interim Final Rule*, 2012, http://www.hhs.gov/ocr/privacy/hipaa/administrative/enforcementrule/hitechenforcementifr.html.

86    Health care IT News Staff, *At a Glance: Stage 2 Final Rule*, August 23, 2012, http://www.healthcareitnews.com/news/glance-stage-2-final-rule.

87    Department of Health and Human Services; Centers for Medicare & Medicaid Services, "Medicare and Medicaid Programs; Electronic Health Record Incentive Program—Stage 2," in *Department of Health and Human Services; Centers for Medicare & Medicaid Services* (2012), 1-672.

88    Congressional Research Service, *Health Information Technology: Promoting Electronic Connectivity in Health care*, April 13, 2005, http://congressionalresearch.com/

RL32858/document.php?study=Health+Information+T echnology+Promoting+Electronic+Connectivity+in+He alth care.

89      Robert Miller, Christopher West, Tiffany Martin Brown, Ida Sim and Chris Ganchoff, "The Value Of Electronic Health Records In Solo Or Small Group Practices," *Health Affairs* 24, no. 5 (September 2005): 1127-1137.

90      U.S. Department of Health & Human Services, *Summary of the HIPAA Privacy Rule*, 2012, http://www.hhs.gov/ ocr/privacy/hipaa/understanding/summary/index.html.

91      Reardon, Thomas R., *Board of Trustees Report 27: Federal Government Investigations of Fraud and Abuse in the Delivery of Health Care Services*, (American Medical Association, 1997).

92      U.S. Department of Health & Human Services, *Health Care Fraud Prevention and Enforcement Efforts Result in Record-Breaking Recoveries Totaling Nearly $4.1 Billion*, February 14, 2012, http://www.hhs.gov/news/ press/2012pres/02/20120214a.html.

93      National Committee for Quality Assurance , *What is HEDIS?* , 2012, http://www.ncqa.org/ HEDISQualityMeasurement/WhatisHEDIS.aspx.

94      AAFP News Staff, *RAC Audits of E/M Services Set to Begin in 15 States*, August 18, 2012, http://www.aafp. org/online/en/home/publications/news/news-now/ practice-professional-issues/20120918racaudits.html.

95      American Hospital Association, *Recovery Audit Contractor (RAC) Program*, 2012, http://www.aha.org/ advocacy-issues/rac/index.shtml.

96      American Academy of Neurology et al, "Letter to Marilyn Tavenner Acting Administrator Centers for Medicare & Medicaid Services," *aan.com*, October 19,

2012, http://www.aan.com/globals/axon/assets/10257.
pdf.

97    Centers for Medicare and Medicaid Services, *Affordable Care Act Update: Implementing Medicare Cost Savings*, August 2, 2010, http://www.cms.gov/apps/docs/ACA-Update-Implementing-Medicare-Costs-Savings.pdf.

98    Joe Cantlupe, *Urologists Follow the Money* , April 12, 2012, http://www.healthleadersmedia.com/page-1/PHY-278893/Urologists-Follow-the-Money.

99    U.S. Department of Health & Human Services, *HITECH Act Enforcement Interim Final Rule*, 2012, http://www.hhs.gov/ocr/privacy/hipaa/administrative/enforcementrule/hitechenforcementifr.html.

100   Jaley Cranford, *Drug Reps: Where Are They Now?*, October 10, 2011, http://platformmagazine.org/2011/12/drug-reps-where-are-they-now/.

101   Pharmaceutical Research and Manufacturers of America, "Code on Interactions with Health care Professionals," *pharma.org*, July 2008, http://www.phrma.org/sites/default/files/369/phrma_marketing_code_2008-1.pdf.

102   Pharmaceutical Research and Manufacturers of America (PhRMA), *Pharmaceutical Research and Manufacturers of America (PhRMA)*, http://www.phrma.org/about/principles-guidelines/code-interactions-health care-professionals.

103   Peter Jones, "Lipids: New Guidelines, Intensive Treatment, and Future Directions," *Texas Heart Institute Journal* 33, no. 2 (2006): 180-183.

104   Beth Smith, Nancy Lee Lee, Elizabeth Haney and Susan Carson, "Drug Class Review: HMG-CoA Reductase Inhibitors (Statins) and Fixed-dose Combination

Products Containing a Statin" (Portland, Oregon: Oregon Health & Science University, 2009).

105 *Therapeutic Interchange and Equivalence: Focus on Antihypertensive Agents Substitution at the Pharmacy Level*, 2012, http://www.medscape.org/viewarticle/416390_4.

106 *Tort*, November 23, 2012, http://en.wikipedia.org/wiki/Tort.

107 Hani, *Andreas Vesalius and Modern Human Anatomy*, 2010, http://explorable.com/andreas-vesalius.html.

108 Jeffrey A Claridge and Timothy C Fabian, "History and Development of Evidence-based Medicine," *Worldn Journal of Surgery*, May 2005: 547-553.

109 Rosenberg WM, Gray JA, Haynes RB, Richardson WS. Sackett DL, "Evidence Based Medicine: What it is and What it Isn't.," *BMJ* 321 (1996): 71.

110 J H Greer, *A Physician in the House* (Chicago: J H Greer, 1897).

111 B Frank Scholl, *Library of Health* (Philadelphia: Historical Publishing Co, 1916).

112 USPSTF Program Office, *U.S. Preventive Services Task Force*, 2012, http://www.uspreventiveservicestaskforce.org/.

113 American Diabetes Association, *Diabetes Care*, January 2012: S11-S63.

114 *Pay for Performance (Health care)*, May 23, 2012, http://en.wikipedia.org/wiki/Pay_for_performance_(health care).

115 American Academy of Family Physicians, *Pay-For-Performance*, 2012, http://www.aafp.org/online/en/home/policy/policies/p/payforperformance.html.

116    Centers for Medicare & Medicaid Services (CMS), "An Introduction to the Medicare EHR Incentive Program for Eligible Professionals," *cms.gov*, 2012, http://www.cms.gov/Regulations-and-Guidance/Legislation/EHRIncentivePrograms/Downloads/Beginners_Guide.pdf.

117    Centers for Medicare and Medicaid Services, *EHR Incentive Programs*, August 27, 2012, http://www.cms.gov/Regulations-and-Guidance/Legislation/EHRIncentivePrograms/index.html.

118    Centers for Medicare & Medicaid Services, *Physician Quality Reporting System*, September 27, 2012, http://www.cms.gov/Medicare/Quality-Initiatives-Patient-Assessment-Instruments/PQRS/index.html.

119    American Medical Association, "2012 Physician Quality Reporting System" (2011).

120    Centers for Medicare and Medicaid Services, *Electronic Prescribing (eRx) Incentive Program*, March 23, 2013, https://www.cms.gov/Medicare/Quality-Initiatives-Patient-Assessment-Instruments/ERxIncentive/Spotlight.html.

121    National Committee for Quality Assurance, "Patient-Centered Medical Home NCQA," *NCQA.org*, 2011, http://www.ncqa.org/Programs/Recognition/PatientCenteredMedicalHomePCMH.aspx.

122    National Committee for Quality Assurance, *Patient-Centered Medical Home*, 2012, http://www.ncqa.org/Programs/Recognition/PatientCenteredMedicalHomePCMH.aspx.

123    National Committee on Quality Assurance, "NCQA PATIENT-CENTERED MEDICAL HOME (PCMH 2011)," *ncqa.org*, January 2011, http://

www.ncqa.org/Portals/0/Programs/Recognition/ PCMH_2011_Pricing_Schedule%282%29.pdf.

124 "Patient-Centered Medical Home Checklist," *ncafp.com*, 2012, www.ncafp.com/files/pcmhChecklist.pdf.pdf.

125 *Accountable Care Organization*, 2012, http://en.wikipedia. org/wiki/Accountable_care_organization.

126 Phillip Longman, *The Best Care Anywhere*, January/ February 2005, http://www.washingtonmonthly.com/ features/2005/0501.longman.html.

127 Office of National Drug Control Policy, *Prescription Drug Abuse*, 2012, http://www.whitehouse.gov/ondcp/ prescription-drug-abuse.

128 Josh Hart, "Slipknot Bassist Paul Gray's Doctor Charged with Manslaughter in Eight Deaths, Band Issue Statement," *Guitar World*, September 6, 2012.

129 Hoggart B. Williamson A, "Pain: a Review of Three Commonly Used Pain Rating Scales.," *Journal of Clinical Nursing* 14, no. 7 (August 2005): 798-804.

130 Drug Safety and Risk Management Advisory Committee, "Acetaminophen Overdose and Liver Injury —Background and Options for Reducing Injury," *fda.gov*, May 29, 2009, http:// www.fda.gov/downloads/AdvisoryCommittees/ CommitteesMeetingMaterials/Drugs/ DrugSafetyandRiskManagementAdvisoryCommittee/ UCM164897.pdf.

131 Jack Brammer, *Bills to Regulate Pain Clinics, Synthetic Drugs Clear House Panel*, February 29, 2012, http://www. kentucky.com/2012/02/29/2089130_house-panel- approves-bills-to.html.

132   Tanya Albert, *Doctor Guilty of Elder Abuse for Undertreating Pain*, July 23, 2001, http://www.ama-assn. org/amednews/2001/07/23/prl20723.htm.

133   Weinman J, Dale J, Newman S. Williams S, "Patient Expectations: What do Primary Care Patients Want from the GP and How Far docs Mccting Expectations Affect Patient Satisfaction?," *Family Practice* 12, no. 2 (1995): 193-201.

134   *Why It's So Important For Physicians To Listen – The Patient's Perspective*, June 11, 2012, http://healthecommunications.wordpress.com/2012/06/11/why-its-so-important-for-physicians-to-listen-the-patients-perspective/.

135   Susan Door Goold and Mack Lipkin, "The Doctor–Patient Relationship," *Journal of General Internal Medicine* 14, no. S1 (January 1999): S26–S33.

136   Indiana State Department of Health, *Local Health Departments–Indiana*, November 17, 2012, http://www.in.gov/isdh/21953.htm.

137   Health Resources and Services Administration Maternal and Child Health Division, *Title V Maternal and Child Health Services Block Grant Program*, 2012, http://mchb.hrsa.gov/programs/titlevgrants/index.html.

# References

Health Resources and Services Administration Maternal and Child Health Division. *Title V Maternal and Child Health Services Block Grant Program.* 2012. http://mchb.hrsa.gov/programs/titlevgrants/index.html.

National Heart Lung and Blood Institute. *What Are the Signs and Symptoms of Pneumonia?* March 1, 2011. http://www.nhlbi.nih.gov/health/health-topics/topics/pnu/signs.html.

Pharmaceutical Research and Manufacturers of America (PhRMA). *Pharmaceutical Research and Manufacturers of America (PhRMA).* http://www.phrma.org/about/principles-guidelines/code-interactions-health care-professionals.

WebMD. *Physician Compensation Report 2011.* 2012. http://www.medscape.com/sites/public/physician-comp/2011.

Æsop. *Æsop's fables, retold by Joseph Jacobs.* New York: P.F. Collier & Son, 1909–14.

123HelpMe.com. *Anarchy.* November 24, 2012. http://www.123helpme.com/view.asp?id=39741.

AAFP News Staff. *RAC Audits of E/M Services Set to Begin in 15 States.* August 18, 2012. http://www.aafp.org/online/

en/home/publications/news/news-now/practice-professional-issues/20120918racaudits.html.

AAMC. *U.S. Medical School Applicants and Students 1982-83 to 2011-12.* AAMC, 2012, 1-5.

Abood, RR. "Cut Pharmaceutical Costs, but Mind the Legal Dangers." *Manag Care*, August 1997: 47-8, 51-4.

*Accountable Care Organization.* 2012. http://en.wikipedia.org/wiki/Accountable_care_organization.

Admi, H, Tzuschinsky O, Herer P, and Lavis P. "Shift work in nursing: Is it really a risk factor for nurses' health and patients' safety?" *Nurse Econ,* July-August 2008.

Albert, Tanya. *Doctor Guilty of Elder Abuse for Undertreating Pain.* July 23, 2001. http://www.ama-assn.org/amednews/2001/07/23/prl20723.htm.

Alemayehu, Berhanu , and Kenneth Warner. "The Lifetime Distribution of Health Care Costs." *Health Services Research* 39, no. 3 (June 2004): 627–642.

Alzolibani, Abdullateef A. "Patient Satisfaction and Expectations of the Quality of Service of University Affiliated Dermatology Clinics." *Journal of Public Health and Epidemiology* 3, no. 2 (February 2011): 61-67.

American Academy of Family Physicians. "Family Physician and Nurse Practitioner Training." *aafp.org.* October 27, 2010. http://www.aafp.org/online/etc/medialib/aafp_org/documents/press/nurse-practicioners/np-training.Par.0001.File.tmp/NP_Info_FP-NPTraining-Compare-4pgs.pdf.

—. *Number of Accredited Programs, Approved First-Year Positions, National Residency Match Program (NRMP) Fill Rate, Actual Fill Rate, and Total Residents for Family Medicine Residency Programs (as of July 2012)* . 2012. http://www.aafp.org/online/en/home/aboutus/specialty/facts/21.html.

—. *Pay-For-Performance*. 2012. http://www.aafp.org/online/en/home/policy/policies/p/payforperformance.html.

American Academy of Neurology et al. "Letter to Marilyn Tavenner Acting Administrator Centers for Medicare & Medicaid Services." *aan.com*. October 19, 2012. http://www.aan.com/globals/axon/assets/10257.pdf.

American Association of Colleges of Osteopathic Medicine. *What Is Osteopathic Medicine?* . 2012. http://www.aacom.org/about/osteomed/pages/default.aspx.

American Cancer Society. *What are the Key Statistics About Breast Cancer?* October 31, 2012. http://www.cancer.org/cancer/breastcancer/detailedguide/breast-cancer-key-statistics.

American Diabetes Association. *Diabetes Care*, January 2012: S11-S63.

American Hospital Association. *Recovery Audit Contractor (RAC) Program*. 2012. http://www.aha.org/advocacy-issues/rac/index.shtml.

American Medical Association. "2012 Physician Quality Reporting System." 2011.

Association of American Medical Colleges. *Medical College Admission Test (MCAT)*. 2012. https://www.aamc.org/students/applying/mcat/.

Blume, Lili. *Are we Really Living Longer? A Closer Look at Life Expectancy Averages*. February 11, 2011. http://www.neuronalstimuli.com/2011/02/are-we-really-living-longer-a-closer-look-at-life-expectancy-averages/.

Brammer, Jack. *Bills to Regulate Pain Clinics, Synthetic Drugs Clear House Panel*. February 29, 2012. http://www.kentucky.com/2012/02/29/2089130_house-panel-approves-bills-to.html.

Bricker & Eckler LLP. *Face-to-Face Encounter With the Patient Required Before Physicians May Certify Eligibility for Home Health Services or Durable Medical Equipment Under Medicare* . 2012. http://www.bricker.com/services/resource-details.aspx?resourceid=592.

*Caffeine Side Effects.* 2012. http://www.drugs.com/sfx/caffeine-side-effects.html.

Cantlupe, Joe. *Urologists Follow the Money* . April 12, 2012. http://www.healthleadersmedia.com/page-1/PHY-278893/Urologists-Follow-the-Money.

Centers for Disease Control and Prevention . *Pertussis (Whooping Cough).* November 15, 2012. http://www.cdc.gov/pertussis/outbreaks.html.

Centers for Disease Control and Prevention. *Vaccines for Children Program (VFC).* August 31, 2012. http://www.cdc.gov/vaccines/programs/vfc/parents/qa-detailed.html.

Centers for Medicare & Medicaid Services (CMS). "An Introduction to the Medicare EHR Incentive Program for Eligible Professionals." *cms.gov.* 2012. http://www.cms.gov/Regulations-and-Guidance/Legislation/EHRIncentivePrograms/Downloads/Beginners_Guide.pdf.

Centers for Medicare & Medicaid Services. *Physician Quality Reporting System.* September 27, 2012. http://www.cms.gov/Medicare/Quality-Initiatives-Patient-Assessment-Instruments/PQRS/index.html.

—. *Physician Self Referral.* March 27, 2012. http://www.cms.gov/Medicare/Fraud-and-Abuse/PhysicianSelfReferral/index.html.

Centers for Medicare and Medicaid Services. "2012 Physician Quality Reporting System (Physician Quality Reporting) Measures List." December 23, 2011.

—. *Acronym List.* 2012. http://www.cms.gov/apps/acronyms/listall.asp?Letter=ALL.

—. *Affordable Care Act Update: Implementing Medicare Cost Savings.* August 2, 2010. http://www.cms.gov/apps/docs/ACA-Update-Implementing-Medicare-Costs-Savings.pdf.

—. *EHR Incentive Programs.* August 27, 2012. http://www.cms.gov/Regulations-and-Guidance/Legislation/EHRIncentivePrograms/index.html.

—. *Electronic Prescribing (eRx) Incentive Program.* March 23, 2013. https://www.cms.gov/Medicare/Quality-Initiatives-Patient-Assessment-Instruments/ERxIncentive/Spotlight.html.

—. *The Nation's Health Care Dollar, Calendar year 2010.* 2012. http://www.cms.gov/Research-Statistics-Data-and-Systems/Statistics-Trends-and-Reports/NationalHealthExpendData/Downloads/PieChartSourcesExpenditures2010.pdf.

Chantrill, Christopher. *Indiana Government Spending Chart.* October 30, 2012. usgovernmentspending.com.

Charles, Sara C. "Coping with a Medical Malpractice Suit." *wjm.* January 2001. www.ewjm.com.

Cheung-Larivee, Karen. *Doctors, Nurses out of Touch with Patient Expectations.* October 26, 2011. http://www.fiercehealthcare.com/story/doctors-nurses-out-touch-patient-expectations/2011-10-26.

Claridge, Jeffrey A, and Timothy C Fabian. "History and Development of Evidence-based Medicine." *Worldn Journal of Surgery*, May 2005: 547-553.

CNN wire staff. *Pediatrician Ordered to Spend Life in Prison for Molesting Patients.* August 26, 2011.

Congressional Research Service. *Health Information Technology: Promoting Electronic Connectivity in Health care.* April 13, 2005. http://congressionalresearch.com/RL32858/document.php?study=Health+Information+Technology+Promoting+Electronic+Connectivity+in+Health care.

Corr, William. *Testimony on Efforts to Combat Health care Fraud and Abuse.* March 4, 2010. http://www.hhs.gov/asl/testify/2010/03/t20100304a.html.

Cranford, Jaley. *Drug Reps: Where Are They Now?* October 10, 2011. http://platformmagazine.org/2011/12/drug-reps-where-are-they-now/.

Dailey, Patricia A. "JCAHO "Forbidden" Abbreviations." *csahq. org.* January 9, 2004. http://www.csahq.org/pdf/bulletin/issue_3/dailey.pdf.

*Dalai Lama Quotes.* 2012. http://www.brainyquote.com/quotes/quotes/d/dalailama158917.html.

Death Penalty Information Center. *Lethal Injection.* 2012. http://www.deathpenaltyinfo.org/lethal-injection-moratorium-executions-ends-after-supreme-court-decision.

Department of Health and Human Services; Centers for Medicare & Medicaid Services. "Medicare and Medicaid Programs; Electronic Health Record Incentive Program—Stage 2." *Department of Health and Human Services; Centers for Medicare & Medicaid Services.* 2012. 1-672.

Dictionary.com. *Job.* November 17, 2012. http://dictionary.reference.com/browse/job?s=t.

Door Goold, Susan, and Mack Lipkin. "The Doctor–Patient Relationship." *Journal of General Internal Medicine* 14, no. S1 (January 1999): S26–S33.

Drug Safety and Risk Management Advisory Committee. "Acetaminophen Overdose and Liver Injury —Background and Options for Reducing Injury." *fda.gov.* May 29, 2009. http://www.fda.gov/downloads/AdvisoryCommittees/ C o m m i t t e e s M e e t i n g M a t e r i a l s / D r u g s / DrugSafetyandRiskManagementAdvisoryCommittee/ UCM164897.pdf.

*Dunning–Kruger effect.* October 31, 2012. http://en.wikipedia. org/wiki/Dunning%E2%80%93Kruger_effect.

*Electronic Health Record.* November 12, 2012. http://en.wikipedia. org/wiki/Electronic_health_record.

Emanuel, EJ. "Cost Savings at the End of Life. What do the Data Show?" *Journal of the American Medical Association* 275, no. 24 (June 1996): 1907-14.

*Evidence-Based Health Care and Systematic Reviews.* November 9, 2012. http://www.cochrane.org/about-us/ evidence-based-health-care.

*Evidence-based Medicine.* August 31, 2012. http://en.wikipedia. org/wiki/Evidence-based_medicine.

Federal Highway Administration. *U.S. Population Living in Urban vs. Rural Areas.* May 6, 2011. http://www.fhwa.dot. gov/planning/census_issues/archives/metropolitan_plan- ning/cps2k.cfm.

Godlee, Fiona, Jane Smith, and Harvey Marcovitch. "Wakefield's Article Linking MMR Vaccine and Autism was Fraudulent." *BMJ,* January 2011.

Goldberg, Charlie. *A Practical Guide to Clinical Medicine.* 2009. http://meded.ucsd.edu/clinicalmed/history.htm.

Greer, J H. *A Physician in the House.* Chicago: J H Greer, 1897.

Hani. *Andreas Vesalius and Modern Human Anatomy.* 2010. http:// explorable.com/andreas-vesalius.html.

Hanson, David J. *Alcohol Problems and Solutions.* 2012. http:// www2.potsdam.edu/hansondj/AlcoholAndHealth.html.

Hart, Josh. "Slipknot Bassist Paul Gray's Doctor Charged with Manslaughter in Eight Deaths, Band Issue Statement." *Guitar World*, September 6, 2012.

Harvard Health Publications. *Coffee Health Risks: For the moderate drinker, coffee is safe says Harvard Women's Health Watch.* August 2004. http://www.health.harvard.edu/press_releases/coffee_health_risk.

Health care IT News Staff. *At a Glance: Stage 2 Final Rule.* August 23, 2012. http://www.healthcareitnews.com/news/glance-stage-2-final-rule.

*History of Copyright Law.* November 10, 2012. http://en.wikipedia.org/wiki/History_of_copyright_law.

*History of Medicine.* November 24, 2012. http://en.wikipedia.org/wiki/History_of_medicine.

History of Medicine Division, National Library of Medicine. *The Hippocratic Oath.* February 7, 2012. http://www.nlm.nih.gov/hmd/greek/greek_oath.html.

Holmes Jr, David R, Jeffrey A Becker, Christopher B Granger, Marion C Lamacher, Robert Lee Page II, and C Sila. "ACCF/AHA 2011 Health Policy Statement on Therapeutic Interchange and Substitution." *American Heart Association Journal*, August 15, 2011.

Humana, Inc. "2011 Annual Report." *corporate-ir.net.* 2012. http://phx.corporate-ir.net/External.File?item=UGFyZW 50SUQ9MTI5MTY4fENoaWxkSUQ9LTF8VHlwZT0 z&t=1.

Illinois Insurance News. *BCBSIL Parent Company's CEO Pay Increase 61% to $12.9 million.* May 15, 2012. http://www.ilhealthagents.com/blog/tag/health-insurance-company-ceo-salaries-2011/#.ULE2_oYhQZY.

IMDb. *Logan's Run.* 2012. http://www.imdb.com/title/tt0074812/.

Indeed. *IT Specialist Salary.* 2012. http://www.indeed.com/salary/IT-Specialist.html.

Indiana State Department of Health. *Local Health Departments–Indiana.* November 17, 2012. http://www.in.gov/isdh/21953.htm.

Isaac Joseph, Deepu G Mathew, Pradeesh Sathyan, and Geetha Vargheese. "The Use of Insects in Forensic Investigations: An Overview on the Scope of Forensic Entomology." *Journal of Forensic Dental Sciences* 3, no. 2 (2011): 89–91.

Jena AB, Seabury S, Lakdawalla D, Chandra A. "Malpractice Risk According to Physician Specialty." *New England Journal of Medicine* 365, no. 7 (August 2011): 629-36.

Jerbert, Mel E, G Scott Brewster, and Mary Lanctot-Herbert. "Ten percent of patients who are allergic to penicillin will have serious reactions if exposed to cephalosporins." *Western Journal of Medicine,* 2000: 341.

Johnson, Caleb. *Church and Religion.* 2012. http://www.mayflowerhistory.com/History/plymoth7.php.

Jones, Peter. "Lipids: New Guidelines, Intensive Treatment, and Future Directions." *Texas Heart Institute Journal* 33, no. 2 (2006): 180-183.

Joszt, Laura. "Top 10 Peeves Doctors Have About Patients." *Physician's Money Digest,* February 22, 2012.

Kazel, Robert. *Do you Tend to Undercode? You're Not Alone .* November 22/24, 2004. http://www.ama-assn.org/amednews/2004/11/22/bil21122.htm.

Kliff, Sarah. *The Average Employer Health Plan Now Costs $15,745, and that's Kind of Good News.* September 11, 2012. http://www.washingtonpost.com/blogs/wonkblog/

wp/2012/09/11/the-average-employer-health-plan-now-costs-15980-and-thats-kind-of-good-news/.

Koppel, Ross. "What do we Know about Medication Errors Made via a CPOE System Versus Those Made via Handwritten Orders?" *Critical Care* 9, no. 5 (August 2005): 427–428.

Kravitz, Richard. "Patient Satisfaction with Health Care Critical Outcome or Trivial Pursuit?" *J Gen Intern Med* 13, no. 4 (April 1998): 280–282.

Kruger, Justin, and David Dunning. "Unskilled and Unaware of It: How Difficulties in Recognizing One's Own." *Journal of Personality and Social Psychology*, 1999: 1121-1134.

L R Burns, R M Andersen and S M Shortell. "Trends in Hospital/Physician Relationships." *Health Affairs* 12, no. 3 (1993): 213-223.

Lawlor, Debbie, George Davey Smith, and Shah Ebrahim. "Commentary: The hormone replacement–coronary heart disease conundrum: is this the death of observational epidemiology?" *International Journal of Epidemiology* 33, no. 3 (2004): 464-467.

Le, Jennifer. "Therapeutic Management of Bronchitis." *American Journal of Managed Care* 11, no. 1 (February 2005).

Legal Information Institute. *Roe v. Wade.* 2012. http://www.law.cornell.edu/supct/html/historics/USSC_CR_0410_0113_ZS.html.

Levine, Meredith. "Tell the Doctor All Your Problems, but Keep it to Less than a Minute." *The New York Times*, June 1, 2004.

Levinson, Daniel. *Testimony on Preventing Health Care Fraud: New Tools and Approaches to Combat Old Challenges.* March 2, 2011. http://www.hhs.gov/asl/testify/2011/03/t20110302i.html.

Longman, Phillip. *The Best Care Anywhere.* January/February 2005. http://www.washingtonmonthly.com/features/2005/0501. longman.html.

Mahomed NN, Liang MH, Cook EF, Daltroy LH, Fortin PR, Fossel AH, Katz JN. "The Importance of Patient Expectations in Predicting Functional Outcomes after Total Joint Arthroplasty." *The Journal of Rheumatology,* June 2002: 1273-9.

Marano, Hara Estroff. *Laughter: The Best Medicine.* June 21, 2005. http://www.psychologytoday.com/articles/200504/ laughter-the-best-medicine.

McCarthy, Robert L. "Health Care Ethics." www.jblearning. com/.../Health%20Care%20Ethics,%203rd%20editio...

McNaughton-Filion L, Chen JS, Norton PG. "The Physician's Appearance." *Family Medicine* 23, no. 3 (March-April 1991): 208-11.

*Medical home.* July 25, 2012. http://en.wikipedia.org/wiki/ Medical_home.

*Medical Research History.* November 17, 2012. http://explorable. com/medical-research-history.html.

Medicare Learning Network. "Evaluation and Management Services Guide." *CMS.gov.* December 2010. https://www. cms.gov/Outreach-and-Education/Medicare-Learning-Network-MLN/MLNProducts/downloads/eval_mgmt_serv_guide-ICN006764.pdf.

Medina, Jennifer. *Jackson's Doctor Is Sentenced to Four Years.* November 29, 2011. http://www.nytimes.com/2011/11/30/ us/michael-jacksons-doctor-sentenced-to-four-years. html?_r=2&adxnnl=1&adxnnlx=1346898879-fewI-JLkVw4Up04vVhLSgDQ&.

Medscape Today News. *Medscape Physician Compensation Report: 2011 Results.* November 17, 2012. http://www.medscape.com/features/slideshow/compensation/2011.

Mehrabian, Albert. *Silent Messages: Implicit Communication of Emotions and Attitudes.* Belmont, CA: Wadsworth, 1981.

MGMA-ACMPE. *Physician Compensation.* 2012. http://www.mgma.com/physcomp/.

Miller, Robert, Christopher West, Tiffany Martin Brown, Ida Sim, and Chris Ganchoff. "The Value Of Electronic Health Records In Solo Or Small Group Practices." *Health Affairs* 24, no. 5 (September 2005): 1127-1137.

Morbidity and Mortality Weekly Report. *Ten Great Public Health Achievements — United States, 1900-1999* . April 1, 1999. http://www.cdc.gov/mmwr/preview/mmwrhtml/00056796.htm.

National Asthma Education and Prevention Program, Third Expert Panel on the Diagnosis and Management of Asthma. "Section 4, Stepwise Approach for Managing Asthma in Youths ≥12 Years of Age and Adults." In *Expert Panel Report 3: Guidelines for the Diagnosis and Management of Asthma*, by Third Expert Panel on the Diagnosis and Management of Asthma National Asthma Education and Prevention Program. Bethesda (MD): National Heart, Lung, and Blood Institute (US), 2007.

National Cholesterol Education Program. *Risk Assessment Tool for Estimating Your 10-year Risk of Having a Heart Attack.* 2012. http://hp2010.nhlbihin.net/atpiii/calculator.asp.

National Committee for Quality Assurance . *What is HEDIS?* . 2012. http://www.ncqa.org/HEDISQualityMeasurement/WhatisHEDIS.aspx.

National Committee for Quality Assurance. *Patient-Centered Medical Home.* 2012. http://www.ncqa.org/Programs/Recognition/PatientCenteredMedicalHomePCMH.aspx.

—. "Patient-Centered Medical Home NCQA." *NCQA.org.* 2011.http://www.ncqa.org/Programs/Recognition/PatientCenteredMedicalHomePCMH.aspx.

National Committee on Quality Assurance. "NCQA PATIENT-CENTERED MEDICAL HOME (PCMH 2011)." *ncqa.org.* January 2011. http://www.ncqa.org/Portals/0/Programs/Recognition/PCMH_2011_Pricing_Schedule%282%29.pdf.

National Heart Lung and Blood Institute. *What Are Coronary Heart Disease Risk Factors?* February 1, 2011. http://www.nhlbi.nih.gov/health/health-topics/topics/hd/.

—. *What Are the Signs and Symptoms of Bronchitis?* May 1, 2009. http://www.nhlbi.nih.gov/health/health-topics/topics/brnchi/signs.html.

Nauert, Rick. *Quality of Psychotherapy Influenced by Office Décor.* June 8, 2011. http://psychcentral.com/news/2011/06/08/quality-of-psychotherapy-influenced-by-office-decor/26766.html.

NHIC Corp. "Modifier Billing Guide." *medicarenhic.com.* June 2011.http://www.medicarenhic.com/providers/pubs/ModifierBillingGuide0611.pdf.

Office of Inspector General, Department of Health and Human Services. "Audit of Selected States' Medicaid Payments for Services Claimed To Have Been Provided to Deceased Beneficiaries." *oig.hhs.gov.* September 26, 2006. https://oig.hhs.gov/oas/reports/region5/50500030.htm.

Office of National Drug Control Policy. *Prescription Drug Abuse.* 2012. http://www.whitehouse.gov/ondcp/prescription-drug-abuse.

*Office Space–1999 Movie Quotes.* http://www.moviequotes.com/ repository.cgi?pg=3&tt=140304.

P.L.224-2003, SEC.83. *Information Maintained by the Office of Code Revision Indiana Legislative Services Agency.* http:// www.in.gov/legislative/ic/2004/title12/ar15/ch14.5.html.

Papazian, Charlie. *The Complete Joy of Homebrewing.* New York: HarperCollins, 2003.

"Patient-Centered Medical Home Checklist." *ncafp.com.* 2012. www.ncafp.com/files/pcmhChecklist.pdf.pdf.

Patrick Conway, M.D. *Statement on The Overutilization of a Typical Antipsychotics in Long-Term Care Settings .* December 5, 2011. http://www.hhs.gov/asl/testify/2011/11/ t20111130a.html.

*Pay for Performance (Health care).* May 23, 2012. http:// en.wikipedia.org/wiki/Pay_for_performance_(health care).

Pharmaceutical Research and Manufacturers of America. "Code on Interactions with Health care Professionals." *pharma. org.* July 2008. http://www.phrma.org/sites/default/ files/369/phrma_marketing_code_2008-1.pdf.

*Physician Quality Measure Reporting.* 2012. http://www.ama-assn.org/ama/pub/physician-resources/clinical-practice-improvement/clinical-quality/physician-quality-reporting-system.page?

*Post Hoc, Propter Hoc–"After the Fact, Therefore Because of the Fact" .* August 7, 2000. http://www.drury.edu/ess/logic/informal/ Post_Hoc__Ergo_Propter.html.

Pounder, Derrick J. "Postmortem Changes and Time of Death." *dundee.ac.uk.* 1995. http://www.dundee.ac.uk/forensic-medicine/notes/timedeath.pdf.

*Primum Non Nocere.* 2012. http://medical-dictionary.thefreedic-tionary.com/Primum+Non+Nocere.

Public Law 111-148. "The Patient Protection and Affordable Care Act." *gpo.gov.* 2010. http://www.gpo.gov/fdsys/pkg/ PLAW-111publ148/html/PLAW-111publ148.htm.

Reardon, Thomas R. *Board of Trustees Report 27: Federal Government Investigations of Fraud and Abuse in the Delivery of Health Care Services.* American Medical Association, 1997.

Rendon, Ruth. "Dentist's Offer to Lower Bill Yields Prostitution Charge." *Houston Chronicle*, August 20, 2004.

Report of the Board of Trustees of the AMA. *Investigations of Fraud and Abuse.* November 17, 2012. mhtml:file://E:\Book References\Investigations of Fraud and Abuse.mht!http:// www.ama-assn.org/ama/pub/physician-resources/legal-topics/regulatory-compliance-topics/health-care-fraud-abuse/investigations-fraud-abuse.page?

Ricciardelli, Michael. *Drug and Alcohol Addiction, Costs and Lack of Care.* October 22, 2012. http://www.healthreformwatch. com/.

Ronald L. Eisenberg, Leonard Berlin. "When Does Malpractice Become Manslaughter?" *American Journal of Roentgenology* 179, no. 2 (August 2012): 331-335.

Rudman, William J PhD, John S Eberhardt III, William Pierce RHIA, and Susan, PhD Hart-Hester. *Health care Fraud and Abuse.* September 29, 2009. http://perspectives.ahima. org/health care-fraud-and-abuse/.

Sackett DL, Rosenberg WM, Gray JA, Haynes RB, Richardson WS. "Evidence Based Medicine: What it is and What it Isn't." *BMJ* 321 (1996): 71.

Saks, Michael J. "Medical Malpractice: Facing Real Problems and Finding Real Solutions." *William and Mary Law Review*, 1994: 1-35.

Sarraille, William A. "Charging for Non-Medicare Patients at Less than the Medicare Rate." *Ocular Surgery News U.S. Edition*, August 2003.

Schneider, Keith. "Dr. Jack Kevorkian Dies at 83; A Doctor Who Helped End Lives." *New York Times*, June 3, 2011.

Scholl, B Frank. *Library of Health*. Philadelphia: Historical Publishing Co, 1916.

Sirkus, Leah, Susan Lukacs, and Amy Branum. *NCHS Data on Pertussis Hospitalizations in Young Children*. January 7, 2010. http://www.cdc.gov/nchs/data/hestat/pertussis/pertussis.htm.

Smith, Beth, Nancy Lee Lee, Elizabeth Haney, and Susan Carson. "Drug Class Review: HMG-CoA Reductase Inhibitors (Statins) and Fixed-dose Combination Products Containing a Statin." Portland, Oregon: Oregon Health & Science University, 2009.

Southwick, John. *Definition of a Profession*. April 1997. http://www.accc.gov.au/content/index.phtml/itemId/277772.

Steven A. Symes, Ph.D., Erin N. Chapman, M.S., Christopher W. Rainwater, M.S., Luis L. Cabo, M.S., and Susan M.T. Myster, Ph.D. "Knife and Saw Toolmark Analysis in Bone: A Manual Designed for the Examination of Criminal Mutilation and Dismemberment." *crime-scene-investigator. net*. December 2010. http://www.crime-scene-investigator. net/KnifeAndSawToolmarkAnalysisInBone.pdf.

The Department of Health and Human Services and The Department of Justice. *Health Care Fraud and Abuse Control Program*. The Department of Health and Human Services and The Department of Justice, 2008.

—. "Health Care Fraud and Abuse Control Program Annual Report For FY 2007." *oig.hhs.gov*. November 2008. https://oig.hhs.gov/publications/docs/hcfac/hcfacreport2007.pdf.

The Free Dictionary. *Allopathy.* 2012. http://medical-dictionary. thefreedictionary.com/allopathy.

*Therapeutic Interchange and Equivalence: Focus on Antihypertensive Agents Substitution at the Pharmacy Level.* 2012. http:// www.medscape.org/viewarticle/416390_4.

Thomas, John. ""Paranoia Strikes Deep": MMR Vaccine and Autism." *Psychiatric Times* 27, no. 3 (2010).

Today's Military. ASV*AB Test.* 2012. http://www.todays-military.com/before-serving-in-the-military/asvab-test?campaign_id=SEM2012:on:google:ASvAB_MEPS-what_is_the_asvab:Broad.

*Tort.* November 23, 2012. http://en.wikipedia.org/wiki/Tort.

Turnham, Hollis. "OBRA '87 Summary." *ncmust.com.* January 23, 2002. http://www.ncmust.com/doclib/OBRA87summary. pdf.

U.S Securities and Exchange Commission. *Ponzi Schemes – Frequently Asked Questions.* 2012. http://www.sec.gov/answers/ponzi.htm.

U.S. Department of Health & Human Services. *Health Care Fraud Prevention and Enforcement Efforts Result in Record-Breaking Recoveries Totaling Nearly $4.1 Billion.* February 14, 2012. http://www.hhs.gov/news/press/2012pres/02/20120214a. html.

—. *HITECH Act Enforcement Interim Final Rule.* 2012. http:// www.hhs.gov/ocr/privacy/hipaa/administrative/enforce-mentrule/hitechenforcementifr.html.

—. *New Tools to Fight Fraud, Strengthen Federal and Private Health Programs, and Protect Consumer and Taxpayer Dollars.* July 26, 2012. http://www.health care.gov/news/factsheets/2012/02/medicare-fraud02142012a.html.

—. *Summary of the HIPAA Privacy Rule.* 2012. http://www.hhs. gov/ocr/privacy/hipaa/understanding/summary/index. html.

U.S. Food and Drug Administration. *FDA and ISMP Launch Campaign to Reduce Medication Mistakes Caused by Unclear Medical Abbreviations.* June 18, 2009. http://www.fda.gov/ NewsEvents/Newsroom/PressAnnouncements/2006/ ucm108671.htm.

*U.S. Health Care Costs.* 2012. http://www.kaiseredu.org/issue-modules/us-health-care-costs/background-brief.aspx.

University of Louisville School of Medicine. *Medschool Admissions.* 2008. http://louisville.edu/medschool/admissions/application-process/pre-med-requirements.html.

US Dept of Health and Human Services; National Institutes of Health; National Heart Lung and Blood Institute. "Guidelines for the Diagnosis and Management of Asthma." 2007.

USPSTF Program Office. *U.S. Preventive Services Task Force.* 2012. http://www.uspreventiveservicestaskforce.org/.

Vonnegut, Kurt. *Harrison Bergeron.* 2012. http://www.enotes. com/harrison-bergeron/summary.

Wafa, Tim. *How the Lack of Prescriptive Technical Granularity in HIPAA Has Compromised Patient Privacy.* DeKalb: North Illinois University Law Review, 2010.

Ward, Marlee. *Your Office Décor Represents Your Image.* http://rxmdmar-ketingsolutions.com/your-office-decor-represents-your-image/.

Weiss, Daniel. *AMA Opposes Giving Pharmacists Prescription Authority.* July 10, 2012. http://www.pharmacytimes.com/ news/AMA-Opposes-Giving-Pharmacists-Prescription-Authority.

Wessel, Lois A. "Nurse Practitioners in Community Health Settings Today." *http://clinicians.org.* February 4, 2005. http://clinicians.org/images/upload/wessel_nurse_practitioners.pdf.

*Why It's So Important For Physicians To Listen – The Patient's Perspective.* June 11, 2012. http://healthecommunications. wordpress.com/2012/06/11/why-its-so-important-for-physicians-to-listen-the-patients-perspective/.

Williams S, Weinman J, Dale J, Newman S. "Patient Expectations: What do Primary Care Patients Want from the GP and How Far does Meeting Expectations Affect Patient Satisfaction?" *Family Practice* 12, no. 2 (1995): 193-201.

Williamson A, Hoggart B. "Pain: a Review of Three Commonly Used Pain Rating Scales." *Journal of Clinical Nursing* 14, no. 7 (August 2005): 798-804.